The Solution to a Better Healthy Life

Philip J. Rushemeza, MD., PhD.

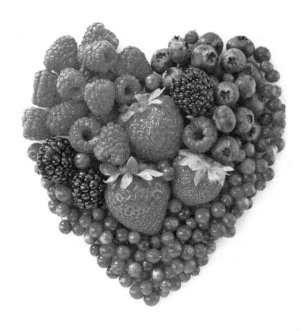

WESTBOW
PRESS®
A DIVISION OF THOMAS NELSON
& ZONDERVAN

The information, ideas, and suggestions in this book are not intended as a substitute for professional medical advice. Before following any suggestions contained in this book, you should consult your personal physician. Neither the author nor the publisher shall be liable or responsible for any loss or damage allegedly arising as a consequence of your use or application of any information or suggestions in this book.

This book is a work of non-fiction. Unless otherwise noted, the author and the publisher make no explicit guarantees as to the accuracy of the information contained in this book and in some cases, names of people and places have been altered to protect their privacy.

WestBow Press books may be ordered through booksellers or by contacting:

WestBow Press
A Division of Thomas Nelson & Zondervan
1663 Liberty Drive
Bloomington, IN 47403
www.westbowpress.com
1 (866) 928-1240

Because of the dynamic nature of the Internet, any web addresses or links contained in this book may have changed since publication and may no longer be valid. The views expressed in this work are solely those of the author and do not necessarily reflect the views of the publisher, and the publisher hereby disclaims any responsibility for them.

Any people depicted in stock imagery provided by Thinkstock are models, and such images are being used for illustrative purposes only.
Certain stock imagery © Thinkstock.

Scripture quotations are from the New Revised Standard Version Bible, copyright © 1989 the Division of Christian Education of the National Council of the Churches of Christ in the United States of America. Used by permission. All rights reserved.

Scripture taken from the King James Version of the Bible.

ISBN: 978-1-5127-8902-7 (sc)
ISBN: 978-1-5127-8903-4 (hc)
ISBN: 978-1-5127-8901-0 (e)
Library of Congress Control Number: 2017908068

Print information available on the last page.

WestBow Press rev. date: 5/23/2017

This book is dedicated to my family, who endured much during my academic quest. I hope that they will treasure it as they continue to live healthy lives.

The Rushemeza family.

CONTENTS

PREFACE

The purpose of this book is to help health professionals, patients, and ordinary people understand and apply medical prevention as a solution for a better healthy lifestyle. It is my humble opinion that good health does not depend on the health care system, physicians, or health workers. Perhaps, instead, it depends on individual choice. It is also true that dependence on physicians alone will not make anyone healthier. Health should be a partnership between physician and the patient.

Many pharmaceutical companies spend a lot of money advertising drugs they want patients to take for particular illnesses, yet people are not cured. Are drugs the solution to better health, or do they create body impairments and dependence?

In this book, I will attempt to examine scientific evidence from many professionals who have dedicated their lives to educating the public on what is best for health. The evidence will show that the solution to better health lies in a change of lifestyle. It is possible that if patients were to follow a God-given diet, practice health awareness, and exercise, there would be no need for most clinic and hospital visits (except for congenital and genetic diseases over which we have no control).

If we continue to depend on health workers for better health, we will continue to depend on drugs, which will soon be like food for daily survival. Health care costs will keep rising and the drug industry will continue to make more drugs, yet people will not be better off.

I argue that world health care should change its course to better health treatment. There is a need for health care workers to educate patients to understand body physiology and teach them preventive measures. Some health workers would like to teach patients to take care of themselves before and after they are sick, but patients do not have time to listen to a physician telling them what to do. Patients need a quick fix on their illness so they can go on with their business. But how can people expect to be well if they do not have time to listen and follow health principles? If we do not change the way we treat them, patients will continue to have problems and treatments may not have great success in most situations.

I also want to emphasize that, although I am not a drug pusher, sometimes there is a need to use drugs. However, it should not be a primary goal of physicians and patients to depend on drugs for curing diseases.

Drugs do not cure diseases; the body cures itself, if it is healthy. The truth is that drugs relieve symptoms and may kill bacteria, but they leave free radicals in the body that may damage the liver, kidneys, lungs, and brain. Taking a drug you don't understand may be gambling with your very life. The side effects of medications can be worse than your pain. Talking to your physician or someone who knows about the medication you're about to put in your mouth may save your life.

The good news is that natural, uncooked foods help to remove free radicals from the liver and blood system. It is said that "cooked food is dead food." This is because cooked foods lose the enzymes that can remove free radicals.

CHAPTER 1
The Leading Cause of Death in the World

Heart disease is the number one cause of premature death in the US and the world. Despite many efforts, it appears that more cases are coming every day, every month, and every year.

What will it take to cure these diseases? So much money has been spent on research, and yet people are not cured. There must be some other way to think about reducing or controlling heart disease among the people in America and the world.

Heart disease does not only affect the Western world; it is a global issue. There was a time when it affected mostly rich people who ate fatty foods, but this is not the case anymore. Such unhealthy foods are found in almost every city and town of the world.

In my experiences traveling the world, I have come to believe that the solution to controlling heart disease will no come from health care workers, lawmakers who fund research, or the modern pharmaceutical industry (Kosuge, Kimura, and Ishikawa, 2006). The solution to this problem is changing diet and lifestyle. High cholesterol, moderate or chronic heart disease, and diabetes are the results of an unhealthy lifestyle. Unhealthy diet, obesity, physical inactivity, and alcohol and tobacco use put people at a higher risk for developing heart disease.

Some types of heart disease can run in the families due to defective genes. We call this situation "congenital." A better lifestyle can reduce the acceleration of such disease even if it cannot be cured. A defective gene can be dominant, meaning that the disease is directly passed down from parent to child, or it may be a recessive gene, meaning the disease jumps generations.

However, defective genes increase in severity with every generation. If one generation started getting the symptoms of heart disease at age fifty, the next generation may get it at forty-five or younger, and the following generation may get the symptoms of the disease at an even younger age. In such cases, we can only control it and but no cure for it.

It' is also true that many genetic disorders can increase the risk of premature heart attack. The most common of these is called familial hypercholesterolemia. This is because of low- level- density protein (LDL) and starts at the time of birth.

It's important to check these heart triggers at birth and throughout your lifetime so you can adjust your lifestyle accordingly. Early diagnosis may help you control the problem, which may affect your overall health (Valensi, Lorgis, and Cottin 2011).

If heart disease isn't congenital, the chance of developing it can be reduced, if not eliminated, in human lives. Individuals can help prevent heart disease by eating a healthy diet, maintaining a healthy weight, exercising regularly, limiting alcohol use, and not smoking, as well as avoiding stress by turning to God, who cares and understands the challenges you face every day in your life.

What Is Coronary Disease?

When we talk about coronary heart disease, it refers to the blood vessels not carrying oxygen properly. If not treated, this can cause muscle and heart tissue damage. Damage to the heart can only be reversed if it's under 70 percent. If the damage is 90 percent or more, it's irreversible. The only thing an individual can do at this point is treat the symptoms and wait for the day when nothing can be done, unless there's a possibility of a heart transplant.

When people come to the doctor after they have severe symptoms, it may be too late in some cases. I remember treating a man who was almost dying of severe coronary heart disease. He had been taking many medications that were causing many other health complications. Changing his lifestyle and diet made him lose weight, and he was able to live four more years. His wife, who didn't get treatment, died of a stroke three years before her husband.

Had this family taken care of themselves when they were younger, they would probably have lived longer. Unfortunately, they started changing their diet and lifestyle too late; the damage was already severe. The solution for this family wasn't in drugs but in a God-given diet and changing their lifestyle.

What Is a Heart Attack?

A heart attack happens when arteries are blocked and they can't carry oxygenated blood to the heart. In some cases, the blockage prevents any oxygen from going to the body tissues. The brain may also suffer from a lack of oxygen and nutrients, which are carried in the blood, resulting in necrosis (tissue death). This causes high blood pressure, chest pain, and fatigue (Jensen, Nyboe, Appleyard, and Schnohr 1991).

Most patients with heart disease live with the belief that it can be cured through surgery or medication. Thus, they're not careful with what they put into their mouths. They drink alcohol, since their physicians have told them that wine is good for the heart. Some use tobacco as a means of relaxation. Nicotine may make people feel good, but the end result of smoking is not good for the heart.

Some other people enjoy eating foods with high cholesterol or calories that the body does not need to exist. The body needs about 2,000 calories a day. In America alone, 4,000 to 6,000 calories are consumed per person per day. The world is getting heavier because of overeating. This doesn't settle well with the heart.

When the body can't handle it anymore, it starts breaking down. These people become new patients, believing that their doctors will fix it all for them. The bad news is that, in most cases of heart disease, if it's an irreversible situation, there's nothing your doctor can do to help you as much as he or she would like to help you get well. You can't blame your doctor. Rather, look at what has brought you to the situation you're suffering from.

What I'm trying to saying here is that prevention is always better than cure. You should not depend on the health care system, but on yourself. As mentioned above, your magic number to reverse tissue damage is below 70 percent. It may continue to be severe if you do nothing about it. It's true that procedures such as bypass surgery and angioplasty can help blood and oxygen flow to the heart more easily. However, these measures are not solutions for better health. The best way is to prevent the damage in the first place if possible (Jensen et al 1991).

Therefore, taking care of yourself before heart trouble comes your way is the best choice. You may think that you're okay now and you can eat and do whatever you want. However, I want you to bear in mind that there are consequences for every bad choice we make in our lives. Whether it's eating, drinking, or smoking, no bad deed will go unpunished. You'll pay, one way or another; there's no exception.

In heart disease, the arteries remain damaged, which means you're more likely to have a heart attack. The condition of your blood vessels will steadily worsen unless you make long-term lifestyle changes. Patients die of complications from heart disease or become permanently disabled. That's why it's so vital to take action to prevent and control this disease.

People who eat a lot of fruit live longer, and non-congenital heart disease isn't one of their main problems. That's why God gave us fruits before sin and vegetables and fruits after sin. When people started eating flesh food, their lives were cut short and full of disease and pain.

Today, the average life span is under seventy years. Some people may say, "Why live longer in this world?" The fact is that God created us for the purpose of service to our fellow people. We should try our best to live healthy lives as much as we can manage it. We should try our best to live free from heart disease so we can continue to serve God and humankind on earth. God wants His people to be healthy: "The Lord will take delight in you and in his Love He will give you new life" (Zephaniah 3:17 GNT).

A good, healthy life comes from God's health principles. Your body forms new cells every day. Without good food and oxygenated blood to carry nutrition and oxygen to every cell and tissue of your body, the tissues will eventually die. Your heart muscles need new cells daily to remain strong and healthy. The heart is an active organ in your body; you need to protect it from overworking itself.

What Causes the Heart to Fail?

The meaning of heart disease is that your heart isn't functioning as it should be. The blood isn't getting to or coming out of the heart chambers. A normal heart works like this: Blood used by the body, which has less oxygen, will enter through the superior vena cava (above the heart) and inferior vena cava (below the heart) in the first chamber, called the right atrium.

Then the heart muscles will squeeze the blood into the lower chamber of the heart, called the right ventricle. The heart muscle will contract again and send blood up to the pulmonary vein, which sends the blood to be oxygenated at the lungs. This is the first stage of blood circulation.

In the second stage, the oxygenated blood from the lungs comes down through the pulmonary artery to the first chamber on the left side of the heart, called the left atrium. The heart contracts again and sends the blood to the left ventricle.

In the final stage, the oxygenated blood from the left ventricle is pushed into the aortic chamber and then out to the rest of the body. The cycle then starts over.

In a normal heart, circulation shouldn't be restricted in any way. It's a cycle that doesn't need any interference. Sometimes the right atrium doesn't open when the blood wants to enter from the superior and inferior vena cava. Where will the blood go? It will have to go back by the help of gravity. This is called right heart failure. Symptoms of it are foot and liver edema (swelling of the lower part of your body). It's also called backflow of blood.

If the blood cannot be squeezed from the heart after it has entered the right atrium, this is because the vessels are not relaxed and open to accommodate the blood flow. Then the heart will be enlarged (cardiomegaly). If the blood cannot enter the second stage from the pulmonary artery, then it goes back to the lungs. This is called left heart failure. A symptom of this is accumulation of fluid in the lungs, which causes you to cough. Let be know that right heart failure can also trigger the left heart failure. In this case the whole heart is not functioning.

Another big problem that mostly affects elderly people is called aortic calcification, meaning that the aorta is not relaxed or able to open because of an accumulation of calcium on its walls. In this case, your doctor will give you calcium channel blockers to relax the aortic muscles so they can contract and the blood can go through that vessel.

Therefore, we should not eat or do anything that will damage the heart. As we shall see in future chapters, animal foods plug the heart vessels, while plant foods open the heart vessels.

As mentioned before, babies can be born with heart disease. This is called congenital heart disease. If people get heart disease later, it is called acquired heart disease. Most heart disease is acquired (Valensi, Lorgis,

Cottin, 2011), caused by overeating or eating unhealthy foods for long periods of time. We bring it on ourselves by not taking care of our diets and living unhealthy lifestyles (Erhardt, Herlitz, Bossaert, 2002).

Congestive Heart Failure

Congestive heart failure affects the second part of the left side of the heart, which can also be triggered by right heart failure. It means the heart fails to pump blood at a normal level. The heart muscle becomes weak. In some cases it is caused by abnormal heart valves that fail to open or may leak blood backward or inside the heart.

When the heart is not able to pump blood because of an obstruction, it has to work extra hard, causing heart palpitations and building inside pressure. If there is too much pressure in the heart, the heart vessels can burst or accumulate blood in the outer layer, which may cause heart congestion or fatigue (Erhardt, Hertlitz, 2002).

Heart Rhythm

A heart rhythm problem is a problem with electrical heart activity. This makes the heart beat too fast or too slow in some cases. If the heart rhythm is too slow or fast, it may make the heart to stop pumping blood. The heart needs a normal and regular beat. Now you can understand why it is not good to drink caffeinated drinks, since they may affect these rhythms (Heart palpitations).

If the rhythm is too fast, the heart may not have time for blood to enter the chambers, so there is not enough blood moving through the heart with each beat. If the heart is too slow, there may not be enough contractions to supply the body with the blood that it needs.

How Do I Know If I Have Heart Disease?

Heart disease and diabetes are silent killers. By the time you feel the symptoms, your body has already been affected. People with heart disease may not know they have it unless they have regular physical checkups. That is why a regular physical checkup is recommended.

Please bear in mind that when you have unusual pain, you should not wait. There is a saying that when you see smoke, there must be fire somewhere. Ignoring symptoms you do not understand may be dangerous to your health.

Once I was driving in Sweden, and I had an appointment to make, so I was in a hurry. However, while I was on the highway, I heard a noise from my front wheel.

Being young and foolish, I kept driving and even put on loud music to drown out the noise. When I got to my destination, I told my friend that I heard a noise from the front left side of my car when I was driving fast. He said he was going to take my car to his own mechanic. When the car was checked, they found only one bolt holding the left front tire on.

You can imagine what would have happened if the tire had fallen off! The lesson I leaned from this situation is not to ignore symptoms. As I mentioned above, where there is a smoke, there must be fire.

Heart Disease in Women

Women generally live longer than men because estrogen provides protection, but heart disease affects women as well. People in developing countries who eat animal fats and exercise less suffer from the same effects as Westerners. Hence, it is very important to eat low-fat diets and exercise (Roe, Messenger, Weintraub, 2010).

Conclusion

At the conclusion of this chapter, we now realize that while some cases of heart disease are congenital, most are acquired due to bad habits or lifestyle. Acquired heart disease can be controlled. People who do not eat processed and refined foods or animal fats suffer less heart disease than those who consume animal products. Heart disease is also a killer in developing countries if they consume excess fats and animal flesh. It is obvious that we are what we eat in many cases.

If we choose what we eat carefully, we will enjoy a good healthy life free from heart disease and diabetes. However, if we eat what our hearts desire, we may end up with these preventable and sometimes unnecessary diseases.

It is also true that if we eat healthy natural foods and less meat, we will be better off and we may not regret that choice. There is chance to live long and happy life free from preventable diseases such as heart disease. Heart disease and diabetes are known as silent killers because by the time you feel the symptoms, your organs are already damaged.

The solution to our health problem is not in medicine or physicians, but rather in each individual examining his/her lifestyle. Ask yourself this question: Is anything I am eating or doing triggering heart disease?" Being aware of the problem will help you reduce death numbers in America and the world.

It is God's purpose that His children be healthy and free from deadly disease. John says, "Beloved, I pray that all may go well with you and you may be in good health just as it is well with your soul" (3 John 1:2 NRSV).

CHAPTER II
Factors in Heart Disease

There are many factors that affect the heart, we need to be aware of the most important ones that can trigger heart disease if not avoided. Heart disease is the leading cause of death in America and the developed world, as mentioned in chapter one of this book. It would appear that it is a disease of rich people who eat anything they like and live any lifestyle they want; at the end it comes back to haunt them. While no one is immune to heart problems, smart lifestyle choices can help us greatly reduce our risk for heart disease (Arad, Goodman, Roth, Newstein, Guerci, 2005)

Heart disease causes heart attacks, stroke, and hypertension (high blood pressure). About 1.2 million people have heart attacks each year in America alone, and about 335,000 die in the emergency room. This is because some of them are not aware of heart disease symptoms or do not check with their doctors as soon as they feel sick. They think it will just go away. Self-reliance is not an American problem: it is a worldwide issue. I have so many friends whom I have difficulty convincing to check their health regularly.

I remember examining a man who was very ill with a heart problem that needed immediate treatment. This man said, "I will be okay. I will go home and rest; then everything will be fine with me." However, his situation did not get better. When he did go to his doctor, he realized how bad it was.

According to the American Heart Association, over 7 million Americans have suffered a heart attack in their lifetime. This is because many people are not aware about the disease until they have symptoms (Kochanek, Murphy, Miniño, Kung, 2009).

Risk Factors for Heart Disease

There are several risk factors for heart disease. Some are controllable and others are not. Uncontrollable risk factors include the following.

Age

Age is a major risk factor for heart disease. More than 83% of people who die from coronary heart disease are 65 or older. This includes women, although women are likely to live longer than men. I have examined many older people with heart problems. You may ask why that happens.

First of all, most elderly people are not very active, they may tend to accumulate cholesterol, and they are on many medications that produce free radicals. Combinations of many medications may not help in elderly people. Another factor is that elderly people often experience more stress and loneliness. That is why if one elderly spouse dies, the other often follows in a short time.

People should be active and eat less animal products when they are young so they can create a pattern of behavior. Remember: practice makes perfect. It is hard to convince the elderly to change the lifestyle they have led for a long time. The behavior developed in youth will most likely be carried on throughout life. Start exercising now and change bad habits so you can benefit from a healthy life.

Gender

Being a man is another factor in heart disease, Psychology supports the notion. Most men do not know how to handle their stress. That is why there are more suicides among men than women. When women are stressed, they often do one of two things to relieve anxiety:

- Call a friend and express how they are feeling.
- Cry out loud, depending on the circumstances.

However, men tend to cook inside their hearts. Men do not easily cry, and always think about how they can overcome whatever is troubling them.

They do not sleep to rest their bodies. Whether rich or poor, men do have it rough.

I have worked as a therapist and pastor, and I have seen and experienced this. So what is the solution to this problem? I suggest that as a man, you do what you can and not force any issues. Remember, if you stress your body, you're either going to trigger heart disease or adopt a lifestyle such as drinking or smoking to help you relax or forget your problem. At the end, nothing is resolved and you affect your health.

Diabetes

Diabetes can also be triggered by stress. If not controlled, it can cause heart disease. Diabetics most likely die of hypertension.

We discussed in chapter one that some cases heart disease is passed from one generation to the next (autosome dominant). It may also jump a generation to another (autosome recessive), and can become more severe. Inherited heart disease is called congenital and is due to defective genes. This is what is called the family history factor. Those with parents or close relatives with heart disease are more likely to develop it themselves.

It is perceived that African Americans, Mexican Americans, American Indians, native Hawaiians, and some Asian Americans have a greater risk compared to Caucasians. This is because of diet and lifestyle.

African Americans and Africans like fried foods. It is true that those foods taste good, but as I always say, not everything that tastes good is good. I am an African American born in Africa. The food I used to eat while I was in Africa is not the same food I enjoyed eating when I lived in Sweden, Norway, and the USA. I ended up paying for it with my health until I changed my diet to mainly fresh fruits and vegetables with more fiber (you will read more about this in later chapters).

Smoking

Smoking is one of the worst enemies of health. It is a lifestyle choice with the end result of death. There is no health benefit in smoking. It is an unnecessary habit, which affects not only you, but the people around you. Many years ago I used to travel on international airplanes that had seats for smokers, and everyone breathed their secondhand smoke. I was very glad when they banned smoking in aircraft. I am thankful that I do not have to smell cigarettes when I travel in airplanes.

Not all cholesterol is bad. You need some amount of cholesterol in your body for the production of energy when the body needs it. However, you have to be aware of how much you need. Too much cholesterol can cause coronary problems and plug your arteries.

If you have ever experienced high blood pressure, you will know what I mean: you feel like a big stone is on your chest. High blood pressure overloads the heart and leaves it thickened and stiff. That is the nature of high blood pressure. It can cause kidney failure, heart attack, and congestive heart failure. The combination of smoking, high cholesterol, and diabetes increases the severity. If not treated, it can claim your life in a short time.

The best solution for this issue is to not smoke or gain too much weight. Your body mass index should be 18-24. Above this range you're asking for trouble at any age.

Having diabetes seriously increases your risk of developing cardiovascular disease. About three-quarters of people with diabetes die from some form of heart or blood vessel disease.

Estrogen protects most women from heart disease until menopause, if they do not have any genetic inheritance of heart disease. However, smoking should be out for them also. It not only increases heart problems, but triggers cancer cells to grow.

Making changes in your lifestyle is a proven method for reducing your risk of heart disease. While there are no guarantees that a heart-healthy lifestyle will keep heart disease away, these changes will certainly improve your health in other ways, such as improving your physical and emotional well-being. Also, because some risk factors are related to others, making changes in one area can benefit other areas (Dohi, Daida, 2010).

Recommendations

Here are some ways you can reduce your risk of heart disease.

Smokers have more than twice the heart attack risk of nonsmokers. Smoking is also the most preventable risk factor. If you smoke, quit. Better never to start smoking at all. Nonsmokers who are exposed to constant smoke (such as living with a spouse who smokes) also have an increased risk, so taking measures to eliminate exposure to smoke is important .

A diet low in cholesterol and saturated and trans fats will help lower cholesterol levels and reduce your risk of heart disease. Regular exercise will also help lower "bad" cholesterol and raise "good" cholesterol. Medications are often needed to reach cholesterol goals before you can take other steps necessary for better health.

About 60 million people in the US. have hypertension or high blood pressure, making it the most common heart disease risk factor. Nearly one in three adults has systolic blood pressure (the upper number) over 140 and/or diastolic blood pressure (the lower number) over 90, which is the definition of hypertension.

Like cholesterol, blood pressure interpretation and treatment should be individualized, taking into account your entire risk profile. Control blood pressure through diet, exercise, weight management, and if needed, medications (Graham, Atar, Borch-Johnsen, 2007)

If not properly controlled, diabetes can contribute to significant heart damage, including heart attacks and death. Control diabetes through a healthy diet, exercise, maintaining a healthy weight, and taking medications as prescribed by your doctor (Clerk, Rattigan, Clark, 2002). However, the best medicine is to control blood sugar by natural means, such as diet and daily exercise.

Exercise has many physiological benefits. It helps to open the insulin receptors. Then the patient gains energy through nutrition, which nourishes the cells. You have to understand that diabetic patients are weak because their body cells are not getting enough nutrition. The cells are starving. Medications can also open the cells, but have side effects. Why not use the natural means that God gave to us freely?

Eat a heart-healthy diet low in salt, saturated fat, trans fat, cholesterol, and refined sugars. Try to increase your intake of foods rich in vitamins and other nutrients, especially antioxidants, which have been proven to lower your risk for heart disease. Also eat plant-based foods such as fruits and vegetables, nuts, and whole grains (Clerk, Rattigan, Clark, 2002).

Gaining weight puts a significant strain on your heart and worsens several other heart disease risk factors such as diabetes, high blood pressure, and high cholesterol and triglycerides. Research is showing that obesity itself increases heart disease risk. By eating right and exercising, you can lose weight and reduce your risk of heart disease (Clerk, Rattigan, Clark, 2002).

During my clinical rotation at West Virginia, the pathologist who taught me clinical pathology was working many hours. Because of stress, he died of a myocardial infarction (MI). Stress can be deadly if not taken care of by a patient and his/her physician. In later chapters, we will discuss more of the effects of stress on the human body.

Some people would argue that smoking relieves stress. I wonder if this is only an excuse to continue smoking? However, the consequences of smoking are far greater than the symptoms of stress. The best thing is to never smoke or quit if you smoke. Cigarette smoking is the most important preventable cause of premature death in the United States. It accounts for more than 440,000 of the more than 2.4 million annual deaths. Cigarette smokers have a higher risk of developing several chronic disorders such as fatty buildups in arteries, several types of cancer, and chronic obstructive pulmonary disease (lung problems) (Jensen, Nyboe, Appleyard, Schnohr, 1991).

Atherosclerosis (buildup of fatty substances in the arteries) is a chief contributor to the high number of deaths from smoking. Many studies detail the evidence that cigarette smoking is a major cause of coronary heart disease, which leads to heart attack. Heart disease is the leading cause of death for people of most ethnicities in the United States, including African Americans, Hispanics, and whites. For American Indians or Alaska Natives and Asians or Pacific Islanders, heart disease is second only to cancer.

Below are the percentages of all deaths caused by heart disease in 2008, listed by ethnicity (Heron, 2012)

Race or Ethnic Group	% of Deaths by Heart Disease
African Americans	24.5
American Indians or Alaska Natives	18.0
Asians or Pacific Islanders	23.2
Hispanics	20.8
Whites	25.1
All	25.0

During 2007–2009, heart disease death rates were highest in the South and lowest in the West. This is because of lifestyle and diet; there can be no other explanation (Graham, Atar, Borch-Johnsen, 2007).

Knowing the warning signs and symptoms of a heart attack is key to preventing death, but many people don't know the signs. In a 2005 survey, most respondents—92%—recognized chest pain as a symptom of a heart attack. Only 27% were aware of all major symptoms and knew to call 911 when someone was having a heart attack (Disparities in Adult Awareness of Heart Attack Warning Signs and Symptoms—14 States, 2005). About 47% of sudden cardiac deaths occur outside a hospital. This suggests that many people with heart disease don't act on early warning signs (State Specific Mortality from Sudden Cardiac Death: United States, 1999; Graham, Atar, Borch-Johnsen, 2007).

Heart attacks have several major warning signs and symptoms:

- Chest pain or discomfort.
- Upper body pain or discomfort in the arms, back, neck, jaw, or upper stomach.
- Shortness of breath.
- Nausea, lightheadedness, or cold sweats (State Specific Mortality from Sudden Cardiac Death: United States, 1999).

High blood pressure, high LDL cholesterol, and smoking are key risk factors for heart disease. About half of Americans (49%) have at least one of these three risk factors (Roger, Lloyd-Jones, 2012). Several other medical conditions and lifestyle choices can also put people at a higher risk for heart disease, including:

- Diabetes
- Overweight and obesity
- Poor diet
- Physical inactivity
- Excessive alcohol use (Roger, Lloyd-Jones, 2012)

Lowering your blood pressure and cholesterol will reduce your risk of dying of heart disease. Here are some tips to protect your heart:

- Follow your doctor's instructions and stay on your medications, if that is the only way to keep you alive.
- Eat a healthy diet that is low in salt, total fat, saturated fat, and cholesterol, and rich in fresh fruits and vegetables. Take a brisk 10-minute walk three times a day, five days a week.
- Don't smoke. If you smoke, quit as soon as possible (Heron, 2012).

A heart attack results from a blockage in the flow of blood to the heart, causing heart cells to die. There are many causes, such as smoking, inactivity, and a diet high in calories, sodium, and saturated fats. Heart attacks are a leading cause of death for both men and women in the United States, and there are several ways to quicken your path to a heart attack. An adult's daily diet should consist of roughly 2,000 calories, with fewer than 1,500 milligrams of sodium, fewer than 16 grams of saturated fat, and fewer than 300 milligrams of cholesterol (World Health Organization, 2008).

Drinking alcohol increases such dangers as alcoholism, breast cancer, suicide and accidents. Also, it's not possible to predict in which people alcoholism will become a problem. Given these and other risks, the American Heart Association cautions people not to start drinking, if they do not already drink alcohol.

Alcohol affects the liver, brain, and other organs of the body. Protect your body organs by not drinking alcohol. The Bible warns, "Wine is a mocker, strong drink is raging; and whosoever is deceived thereby is not wise" (Proverbs 20:1 KJV). There is no wisdom in drinking alcohol. It causes liver damage and also causes brain cells to die. It impairs judgment by affecting the frontal lobe of your brain. You wonder who would want such a drink. That is why the word of God says "whosoever drinks wine is not wise." Yet you hear some health professionals say wine is good for your heart. Are these people above God's wisdom? Think about that.

Conclusion

Heart disease risk factors are more controllable than you think, if you choose to change your lifestyle. Some risk factors for heart disease are genetic, but the majority of cases of heart disease are caused by lifestyle.

A good example is that people in America have higher chances of contracting heart disease and diabetes triggered by lifestyle. I am not saying there are no health problems in Africa, Asia, and South America; heart disease and diabetes exist on every continent. But, you may ask yourself, what makes Africa and America different? The studies clearly show that diet and lifestyle have a whole lot to do with heart disease and diabetes.

Some eat everything their hearts desire, while others have less and eat less refined foods. People in Africa and the rest of the developing world would live longer if it were not for poverty and less nutritional foods. Therefore, some people die from overeating and others die from starvation. Let me be clear that heart disease does not discriminate; it does not matter where you live or what you do in life. Even if you live on the moon or Jupiter, a lifestyle of eating badly, smoking, and drinking will lead you to an early grave from heart disease or cancer. The solution to these problems is to avoid putting bad things into your body and exercise to reduce stress and toxicity.

Those of us who are given this health knowledge ought to set an example in everything we do. It is not good for a physician to tell a patient not to smoke or drink while he/she is a smoker or drinks alcohol. The same applies to foods and other bad lifestyle elements.

The argument has been made that alcohol is good for the body. In some cases, it is true that wine may have some health benefits. However, why not drink grape juice and other fruit juices, which have even better benefits for your body? Why drink alcohol, which has side effects on the heart and mind?

The Bible says, "Do not drink wine or intoxicating drink, you nor your sons with you, when you enter in the tent of meeting, that you may not die, it is a statute forever throughout your generation. You are to distinguish between the holy and the common, and between the unclean and the clean" (Leviticus 10: 9-10 NRSV).

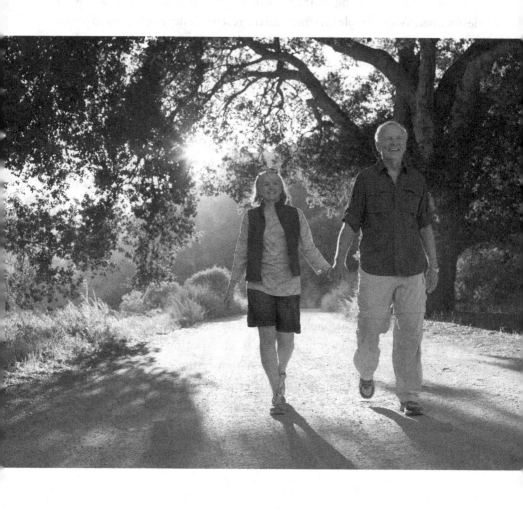

CHAPTER III

Effects of Caffeine on the Heart and Mind

Coffee is considered by many people to be a recreational drink. It makes people feel good, as does eating chocolate. They both have caffeine. There are some cultures where every visitor is offered a cup of coffee as a sign of welcome in the home or when having a special conversation. Some people say they cannot live without coffee every morning. Others have pots of coffee even at work. It is an addictive substance, yet people do not take the time to understand how it affects their lives. In a way, caffeine has controlled their existence, and if they stop drinking coffee, it will cause withdrawal effects.

There is no concrete scientific evidence to support the effects of caffeine on memory. Findings are inconsistent, but some evidence shows that many effects of caffeine impair short-term and working memory instead of helping, as it has been thought.

As a medical doctor, I know for sure that coffee affects the heart as well as the mind. There are also studies suggesting that coffee causes stomach cancer. If you do not believe me, ask yourself why coffee changes mood? and why people tremble and have headaches when they go without it?. This is because of the caffeine in the coffee.

There is a research consensus indicating an inhibitory effect, reducing the capacity of short-term memory and working memory. This is because coffee affects the nerves. It has nothing to do with increasing or reducing memory. In fact, it can impair the mind. This is because drinking coffee can damage your sleep cycle and affect serotonin (Angelucci, Cesário, Hiroi, Rosalen, Da Cunha, 2002).

Effects of Caffeine on the Human Body

It stimulates the central nervous system.

- It releases free fatty acids from adipose (fatty) tissue.
- It affects the kidneys, increasing urination, which can lead to dehydration (Angelucci, Cesário, Hiroi, Rosalen, Da Cunha, 2002).

Caffeine is found in coffee, tea, soft drinks, chocolate, and some nuts (cocoa). Whether caffeine intake improves memory or not, there is a high risk of coronary heart disease among people who drink caffeine.

Caffeine-habituated individuals can experience "caffeine withdrawal" 12–24 hours after the last dose of caffeine. It resolves within 24–48 hours. The most prominent symptom is headache. They can also feel anxiety, fatigue, drowsiness, and depression (Warburton, Bersellinni, Sweeney, 2001).

Caffeine's effects on memory were also investigated in the auditory system. The Auditory-Verbal Learning Test is a memory test that assesses recall of lists of words on single and multiple trials given through the subjects' auditory system. Caffeine subjects recalled fewer words than did control subjects, and caffeine subjects showed a greater deficit in recalling the middle- to end-portions of the lists (Terry, Phifer, 1986).

Caffeine has been thought to have some benefits when testing working memory. The idea was that, if caffeine were present in one's system, then one would be less likely to experience tip of the tongue effect, or the feeling of knowing a familiar word but not being able to immediately recall it. Previous research suggested that the tip of the tongue phenomenon can be corrected for with the use of caffeine, and that caffeine could help one to more quickly retrieve the word they are looking for. However, current research refutes previous research, finding evidence for priming a phonological loop within the working memory as opposed to caffeine enhancing capacity (Terry, Phifer, 1986). When attempting to comprise tip of the tongue effects, subjects were primed with similar-sounding words to the target word; as a result of the priming, the target word was reached faster regardless of caffeine intake (Lesk, Womble, 2004).

Short-term memory has been thought to be influenced differently throughout the day when caffeine has been ingested; in the morning, performance will be different than at the end of the day. Three groups (low, medium, and high caffeine intake) were compared during four daytime hours. People with low caffeine intake had decreased performance later in the day, compared to the other groups. These results are interesting but do not conclusively determine that caffeine impairs or improves short-term memory compared to a control group (Mitchell, 1992).

Coffee is a stimulant. It may not stimulate the mind, but it affects the neurotransmitters. That is why this research is not conclusive. In order to maintain the same effect of stimulant, one has to keep drinking coffee all the time; however, consuming so much caffeine may not be good for the heart.

The firing of neurons will work well when they can fire and act in a normal space without being forced to act by other substances. When caffeine controls the body, in order to function the same way, you will need to keep consuming the caffeine. This is called addiction to caffeine.

When studying the effects of this or any drug, potential ethical restraints on human study procedures lead researchers to conduct studies involving animal subjects in addition to human subjects (Warburton, Bersellinni, Sweeney, 2001). Researchers have found that long-term consumption of low-dose caffeine slowed hippocampus-dependent learning and impaired long-term memory in mice. Caffeine consumption for four weeks also significantly reduced hippocampal neurogenesis compared to controls during the experiment. This may be because caffeine impairs the neurotransmitters. The conclusion was that long-term consumption of caffeine could inhibit hippocampus-dependent learning and memory partially through inhibition of hippocampal neurogenesis (Hameleers, Van Boxtel, Hogervorst, Riedel, Houx, Buntinx, Jolles, 2000).

Let us discuss the hippocampus and how it works with the mind. The hippocampus is located in the front lobe of the brain. This is where new memory is stored in the short term before it can be stored in a long-term memory part of the brain. I would argue that caffeine does not add or enhance new memories. However, since caffeine is a stimulant substance, it may enhance firing of the neurons temporarily. I say temporarily because in order to get the same effect, you need to keep adding the fuel of caffeine to your system.

Positive effects of caffeine on long-term memory have been shown in a study analyzing habitual caffeine intake of coffee or tea in addition to consuming other substances. Their effect on cognitive processes was observed by performing numerous cognitive tasks. Words were presented and delayed recall was measured. Increased delayed recall was demonstrated by individuals with moderate to high habitual caffeine intake (mean 710 mg/week) as more words were successfully recalled compared to those with low habitual caffeine intake (mean 178 mg/week) (Hameleers, Van Boxtel, Hogervorst, Riedel, Houx, Buntinx, Jolles, 2000).

Therefore, improved performance in long-term memory was shown with increased habitual caffeine intake due to better storage or retrieval. A similar study assessing effects of caffeine on cognition and mood resulted in improved delayed recall with caffeine intake. A dose-response relationship was seen as individuals were able to recall more words after a period of time with increased caffeine (Jolles, 2000).

Improvement of long-term memory with caffeine intake was also seen in a study using rats and a water maze. In this study, completion of training sessions prior to performing numerous trials in finding a platform in the water maze was observed. There was no effect of caffeine consumption before the training sessions; however, a greater effect was seen at a low dosage immediately afterward. In other words, the rats were able to find the platform faster when caffeine was consumed after the training sessions rather than before. This implies that memory acquisition was not affected, while increases in memory retention were (Mayo Clinic, retrieved 2012-10-15).

Caffeine has also been shown to have negative effects on long-term memory, in particular, impairment during selected tasks. In a study with mice, a step-through passive-avoidance task was used, and the ability to remember the task was assessed. Caffeine was given before the task in varying doses, with low doses to start (11.55 mg/kg) and a higher dose in the end (92.4 mg/kg). To put that in perspective, one 8 oz cup of coffee contains 95–200 mg of caffeine. An apparatus including a box with a light was connected to a dark box with an electric floor. When the mice entered the dark box, a shock was released from the floor. The next day, the mice entered the apparatus again and completed the same task. Subjects that did not enter the dark box for 180 seconds were thought to have put the task in long-term memory, remembering the assignment from the previous day. However, caffeine administered at higher doses resulted in decreased retention time of the task from 180 seconds to 105 seconds. Lower doses of caffeine had little to no effect on retention time (Warburton, Bersellinni, Sweeney, 2001)

Therefore, in this study linear regression analysis showed that higher doses of caffeine impaired long-term memory, suggesting a dose-response relationship between caffeine intake and retention time. Ultimately, long-term memory and caffeine intake display varying results, in human as well as animal subjects (Herz, 1999).

Some studies have shown that caffeine intake has no effect on long-term memory. This was expressed in a study where either caffeine or a placebo was assigned to several subjects at two different times. Some subjects received caffeine first, while others received a placebo. All participants were shown a word list that would eventually be tested. Two days later, the same process was repeated, with random distribution of the two substances. This was also observed in a study involving the assessment of delayed recall using a verbal memory test. Two studies were completed using different control drinks containing caffeine (Warburton, Bersellinni, Sweeney, 2001). Caffeine's effects appear to be detrimental to short-term memory, working memory included, whereas the effects are somewhat positive for memory over the long term (for example, you remember something better many days later if you drank caffeine during encoding as well as retrieval, as opposed to no caffeine). Many of the effects reported were for subjects who were not regular caffeine consumers (Bernstein, Carroll, Dean, Crosby, Perwien, Benowitz, 1998). Regular consumers of caffeine, on the other hand, showed only positive effects when it came to memory tasks. An important factor to consider is that there was fairly wide-range daily caffeine consumption previous to the study, and this could have had a significant effect on performance of the task because not everyone is at the same baseline (Van Boxtel, Schmitt, 2004).

Effects of Caffeine by Age and Sex

Another study used a much larger subject pool and found that age-related differences were quite minimal for intentional memory, but that over the long term, regular caffeine consumption was fairly beneficial to younger subjects (Schmitt, 2003).

As previously stated, the most pronounced effect of caffeine on memory appears to be on middle-aged subjects (26-64). None of the studies provide reasoning for why this group would be most affected, but one could hypothesize that because of cognitive decline due to age, caffeine has a powerful effect on brain chemistry (although this would suggest the older the person, the stronger the effect of caffeine). Furthermore, this age group is most likely to be the largest consumer of caffeine. The main studies reporting this show that at low, acute doses of caffeine consumption, working memory is only slightly affected for those in this age group, while no effect is observed for younger or older subjects. The authors conclude that larger doses may be needed to produce results that are supported by previous literature, and this is an avenue for further research. Furthermore, it is argued that consumption of caffeine generally aids cognitive performance for this age group, as long one does not exceed the recommended dose of 300 mg per day (Ryan, Hatfield, Hofstetter, 2002).

In older adults, memory is typically best in the morning and gradually declines over the day. Those who consumed caffeine in the morning showed much better memory, both short-term and long-term, than those who consumed a placebo, especially in late afternoon, when memory and attention may be most crucial to daily functioning for the elderly. This is further supported by a study which showed that adults over the age of 65 who regularly consume caffeine in the morning are much more alert and function at a higher cognitive level throughout the day.

It is beneficial for older adults to regularly consume average doses of caffeine in the morning to boost cognitive performance and alertness in the afternoon. Again, one should not exceed the recommended dose of about 300 mg per day; otherwise memory performance declines due to over-consumption (Erikson, Hager, Houseworth, Dungan, Petros, 1985).

Sex differences have not been thoroughly covered in the literature concerning caffeine's effect on memory. Since most studies do not report significant sex differences in this area of memory study, it is reasonable to assume that there is not strong evidence to support sex differences in caffeine's effect on memory (Richardson, Elliman, Rogers, 1995). Further specific research into sex differences would be needed to fully understand the impacts of this popular drug on its users.

However, some studies provide support for the idea that caffeine has different effects on males versus females when related to memory. These differences can be seen through a number of memory types (short-term, long-term, etc.), with various theories accounting for these differing effects (Arnold, Petros, Beckwith, Gorman, 1987)

Caffeine has been shown to have an impairing effect on females (but not males) in a word-list test of short-term memory. One prevailing theory that aims to explain this sex difference identifies estrogen levels in the body as an important factor relating to caffeine's effect on memory performance (Richardson, Elliman, Rogers, 1995). The female menstrual cycle (which influences overall estrogen levels in the body) may play a role in modifying the effect of caffeine on memory. Following this theory, researchers tested females within the first five days of their menstrual cycle and found that caffeine had a facilitative effect on female performance on a short-term memory test (Bernstein, Carroll, Dean, Crosby, Perwien, Benowitz, 1998).

A particular finding in this study relating to male memory performance revealed that at a lower dose, caffeine had an impairing effect, but at higher doses, no impairment was shown. It is also interesting to note that differing speeds of testing (words delivered slowly or quickly) in males served as a modifying factor on the effect of caffeine: higher doses aided in recall with faster presentation of words, and lower doses aided in recall with slower presentation of words.

These findings are only based on a small set of data collected from selective studies on this topic, so further research in this area would be needed to gain a more clear understanding of caffeine's differing effects on male and female short-term memory (Bernstein, Carroll, Dean, Crosby, Perwien, Benowitz, 1998).

Effects of Caffeine Withdrawal on the Body

Caffeine withdrawal has been known about for over a hundred years. However, there are still many unknowns that exist, because only within the last decade has it been researched scientifically. As of this point in time, there is no known correlation between caffeine withdrawal and an effect on memory. There are many potential reasons for the lack of conclusions made about this issue.

The main speculation is that since caffeine affects many parts of the central nervous system, there is more than one mechanism that is activated by caffeine. It would thus require the examination of multiple activation pathways in order to determine caffeine's specific effect on the nervous system and consequently memory (White, Lincoln, Pearce, Reeb, Vaida, 1980). Even though there is no direct evidence that caffeine withdrawal impacts memory, there are many other connections made that provide some insight into what memory effects are possible. For example, there is evidence to show that attention decreases when experiencing caffeine withdrawal. A study had school-age children who were regular caffeine users go 24 hours without caffeine consumption, and the results showed a decrease in performance on reaction time of a task that required attention.

Studies have also shown that regular caffeine users experience headaches and fatigue during withdrawal. One study had a group of regular caffeine users divided into three groups. Each group was designated an amount of time to avoid caffeinated products: 1.5 hours, 13 hours, or 7 days. The study found that, to varying degrees, all participants experienced an increase in fatigue, drowsiness, and headaches.

A third study found that among a group of participants receiving a placebo, anxiety was experienced by participants who had prior caffeine use. This would imply that participants would also experience a deficit in memory capabilities because attention and alertness positively impact the amount of information that can be stored in both short- and long-term memory, and anxiety would be a detriment to memory retention (Richardson, Elliman, Rogers, 1995).

There is also existing evidence that reflects on the duration of the caffeine avoidance period in relation to the significance of the withdrawal symptoms. In the study previously mentioned, the strongest withdrawal effects were seen among participants who underwent a 13-hour avoidance period, followed by the 7-day avoidance group. This would imply that memory effects would be at their strongest around the 13-hour mark and would continue to be affected for the following days. Memory would not be affected, however, within the first few hours.

This appears valid, considering most daily caffeine users need to consume caffeine shortly after awaking from sleep. For example, coffee drinkers were given either caffeine or a placebo after overnight caffeine abstinence. The study showed that regular coffee drinkers became less alert and more anxious than non-coffee drinkers when receiving the placebo. To coincide with this finding, another study found a dose-related improvement in cognitive performance for daily caffeine users. This means that coffee drinkers experience the same positive effects every day they consume coffee (Rogers, Heatherley, Hayward, Seers, Hill, Kane, 2005).

Does administration of caffeine to withdrawal participants reverse the effects? The answer to this question is inconclusive, but there have been some suggestions. One study that evaluated a caffeinated taurine drink found that all participants experienced an increase in informational processing after consuming caffeine, regardless if there was a withdrawal period. This would imply that caffeine has the same effect despite differences in withdrawal symptoms.

However, another study found that caffeine could improve cognitive performance with participants who experienced both long- and short-term caffeine avoidance, but was ineffective with participants who had not experienced avoidance. Yet a third study found that over-consumption of caffeine produced virtually no positive side effects for caffeine non-users (Van Boxtel, Schmitt, 2004).

Conclusion

As numerous studies have shown above, caffeine is a stimulant substance. It may help with firing of the neurotransmitters. It does not increase or reduce memories. Caffeine affects the heart and increases heart palpitations. Even though it may have some temporary benefits, caffeine is not the best for your heart and mind in the long run. In fact, there are some studies linking caffeine to stomach cancer.

There are other methods to improve memory without consuming caffeine. Some people may want to enjoy today's pleasure and suffer tomorrow; we call this a choice. However, running, or any other exercise in the open air, gives you the same benefit of stimulating memory, due to oxygen flow in the brain. It is also helpful to eat healthy foods such as apples, watermelon, and uncooked vegetables. These foods take away toxicity from the GI and blood, and they nourish the brain as well as the whole body. Beans can be a source of dopamine to nourish the brain as well.

Your body should not be intoxicated with caffeine, nicotine, or alcohol.

It is bought by the priceless blood of Jesus your Savior. When man refuses to follow God's way, the body is destroyed and becomes dependent on substances that affect the heart and nervous system.

I would, therefore, conclude that if you depend on caffeine to wake you up, you will depend on caffeine all of your life. Bear in mind that it will cause your heart to work extra hard and affect your resting state. You will not have complete sleep with a full cycle of rest. It may even cause anxiety. Too much firing of the neurotransmitters (which carry information in the brain) may affect judgment and cause an anxious state of mind.

I recommend that you avoid caffeine so your body and mind can rest and reset your mind and body in a normal way without being forced to function. Caffeine may feel good today, but it requires payback tomorrow.

CHAPTER IV
Effects of Stress on the Human Body

Stress is the body's reaction to any change that requires an adjustment or response. The body reacts to these changes with physical, mental, and emotional responses. Stress is a normal part of life. Many events that happen to you and around you—and many things that you do yourself—put stress on your body.

Stress is like an acid in the body. It causes anxiety and affects neurotransmitters and brain function. It causes heart palpitations and forces the heart to work hard to find sources of energy if the liver does not have enough glucose to supply for action potential. That is the reason why stress triggers the release of cholesterol from the body storage.

Stress increases cholesterol in the body. For diabetics and those with heart disease, it makes it worse. You may experience stress from your environment, your body, and your thoughts. The human body is designed to experience stress and react to it. Stress can be positive, keeping us alert and ready to avoid danger. Stress becomes negative when a person faces continuous challenges without relief or relaxation between challenges. The person becomes overworked and stress-related tension builds.

Stress that continues without relief can lead to a condition called a negative stress reaction. Distress can lead to physical symptoms including headaches, upset stomach, elevated blood pressure, chest pain, and problems sleeping. Research suggests that stress also can bring on or worsen certain symptoms or diseases.

Stress also becomes harmful when people use alcohol, tobacco, or drugs to try and relieve their stress. Unfortunately, instead of relieving the stress and returning the body to a relaxed state, these substances tend to keep the body in a stressed state and cause more problems. Forty-three percent of all adults suffer adverse health effects from stress (Steptoe, Kivimäki, 2012).

Complications of Stress

Rates of heart attack and sudden death have been shown to increase significantly following the acute stress of natural disasters like hurricanes, earthquakes, and tsunamis, and as a consequence of any severe stressor that evokes "fight or flight" responses (Rosenman, 1995). Coronary heart disease is also much more common in individuals subjected to chronic stress, and recent research has focused on how to identify and prevent this growing problem, particularly with respect to job stress.

In many instances, we create our own stress that contributes to coronary disease through smoking and other bad habits or because of dangerous traits like excess anger, hostility, aggressiveness, time urgency, inappropriate competitiveness, and preoccupation with work (Steptoe, Kivimäki, 2012). These are characteristic of Type A coronary-prone behavior, now recognized to be as significant a risk factor for heart attacks and coronary events as cigarette consumption, elevated cholesterol, and blood pressure. While Type A behavior can also increase the likelihood of these standard risk factors, its strong correlation with coronary heart disease persists even when these influences have been excluded (Steptoe, Kivimäki, 2012).

High levels of cortisol, the so-called stress hormone, have been associated with cardiovascular disease in some studies, but not in others. This may be because measuring cortisol in blood or saliva at one point in time may pick up acute stress, but it fails to account for long-term stress. Dutch researchers assessed cortisol levels over several months by analyzing scalp hair samples and gathered self-reported data about coronary heart disease, stroke, peripheral artery disease, type 2 diabetes, lung disease, cancer and osteoporosis. Compared with those in the lowest quarter for cortisol, those in the highest quarter had about three times the risk of cardiovascular disease and diabetes. There was no association between cortisol levels and risk of lung disease, cancer, or osteoporosis (O'Connor, Brady, Brooks, 2010).

Cholesterol is an essential component that repairs body cells. If extra cholesterol is not efficiently removed from the bloodstream, however, it can lead to serious conditions, such as coronary heart disease and stroke. A buildup of cholesterol can be linked, in part, to stress. During stress, primitive instincts prepare the body for flight or fight. As a protection mechanism, the body triggers the generation of two hormones, cortisol and adrenaline, that increase blood flow to the brain and act as stimuli to release more energy, but also trigger the production of cholesterol. Cortisol produces more sugar in order to provide the body with instant energy to tackle the stressful situation. The high sugar levels, however, often are not used up by the body and eventually are converted to fatty acids and cholesterol.

The effects of high cholesterol in the bloodstream are seen very late, often years after the cholesterol levels have started rising. With an increase in low-density lipoprotein (LDL, also known as bad cholesterol) and a decrease in high-density lipoprotein (HDL, also known as good cholesterol), cholesterol deposits start accumulating in the walls of arteries and other organs. This can lead to diseases such as angina, heart attack, stroke, coronary disease, and peripheral artery disease. Many of these diseases are life-threatening if left untreated.

High cholesterol can be detected by a simple blood test, the lipid profile. This test should be done at regular intervals, usually annually, to ensure that any increase of cholesterol is detected early. If the cholesterol levels are high for a prolonged period, a doctor might order specific tests to diagnose other disorders caused by this condition.

Stress can push people toward unhealthy eating habits and lifestyles, such as smoking, drinking, and a diet that contributes to high cholesterol. Some people use stress as an excuse to continue smoking without considering the long-term effects on the heart and lungs. However, living a healthy lifestyle can prevent stress and high cholesterol. Avoid smoking and drinking alcohol; exercise regularly to combat a sedentary life and obesity; reduce body fat by eating fibrous foods with low oil content, such as leafy vegetables; eat a high-fruit diet; and practice yoga or meditation to relax and relieve your mind of stress.

How to Increase Dopamine and Relieve Stress

The dopamine naturally produced by your brain makes you feel good. You get a rush of dopamine in response to pleasurable activities like food or sex. On the other hand, without enough dopamine, you may feel sluggish, depressed, and uninterested in life.

It is better to increase this hormone through natural foods instead of chemicals. Almonds, avocados, bananas, low-fat dairy, meat and poultry, lima beans, sesame seeds, and pumpkin seeds may all help your body to produce more dopamine, as can soy products (like tofu, etc.). However, many dairy and meat products are high in calories and fat, so use dairy with caution and monitor your caloric intake with this high-dopamine diet. Dopamine is easy to oxidize, and antioxidants may reduce free radical damage to the brain cells that produce dopamine. Many fruits and vegetables are rich in antioxidants, including greens, orange vegetables and fruits, asparagus, broccoli, and beets.

Avoid food that inhibits brain function; such foods may include refined packaged foods, refined white flour, cholesterol, caffeine, and saturated fats. When you get addicted to something (even coffee!), your dopamine receptors need more and more to trigger. Junk foods are addictive too! You ever wonder why eating too much junk food makes us feel groggy? It inhibits dopamine production, making us feel sluggish and unable to find pleasure in the little things. Sticking to fruits, veggies, low-fat dairy, and meats is a surefire way to stay on top of your mental game. Exercise increases blood calcium, which stimulates dopamine production and uptake in your brain. Try 30 to 60 minutes of walking, swimming, or jogging to jump-start your dopamine levels.

One of the best ways to feel energized and ready to tackle the day is to get plenty of sleep. Dopamine has been tied to feelings of wakefulness, so in order to get that wakeful feeling, get seven or eight hours of sleep a night.

Dopamine is all about pleasure; it's one hedonistic brain chemical, that's for sure. Luckily, all you have to do is train your brain. The problem is that most people want a quick and easy fix, which is not necessarily effective. The brain wants to be treated slowly but surely. In other words, if the body feels tired, obey it; do not force it to keep working. If you force the body to keep working, you may break it. Many people force it with drugs or caffeine to keep the body awake. The brain does not like this. You may end up paying for your bad behaviors.

If you're really struggling to focus on tasks and experiencing hyperactivity, your doctor can prescribe psychostimulants like Ritalin to stimulate dopamine production in your brain. However, it should not be a habit, as it may affect your sleep. Low dopamine levels are also sometimes associated with depression. If you need a quick fix for depression, you can talk to your doctor about starting an antidepressant. However, it is best to increase dopamine through natural foods, rest, exercise, and other natural means instead of drugs.

The best way is to know what you're doing and what you want to achieve from the treatment. If natural means don't work to relieve symptoms of low energy, you have to find the root of your problem. Treating symptoms through medication alone may not be a solution to your health problem. Find the problem and deal with it is the best way.

You do not want to increase dopamine levels too much through medication; you may turn from depression to schizophrenia symptoms. People with conditions like schizophrenia actually produce too much dopamine. Doctors treat conditions like these with antipsychotics, which suppress dopamine production .Many opioids, methamphetamine, and illegal drugs can increase dopamine production. However, these drugs come with a marked risk for addiction, and they can disrupt the way that your body naturally produces dopamine. You can end up feeling depleted, hungry, depressed, and even suicidal after taking opioids or methamphetamine. You're disrupting your chemical balance—it's like giving yourself a mental illness. So don't do it. It may make you feel good, but the results affect your heart and brain health all together. It is never good for you.

The Bible tells us that a happy heart works as medicine, but the sorrowful heart dries the bone (Proverbs 17:22). It is true that as long as we live in this world, we will have problems, which may affect our health. God in His love has provided solutions for His children. We must trust in Him to help us in our troubles (Matthew 11:28). He calls us to bring all of our troubles to Him and He will help us. As Jesus depended on His heavenly father for strength, we need to depend on Him also. We need to pray and look to our heavenly father as Jesus did.

If you let stress take over your life, it may affect your health, and you can build cholesterol in your body. The National Institutes of Health recommend the following methods of stress management: listening to music, practicing yoga, meditation, and eating a low-fat diet with good fiber content. Visit a psychotherapist if the stress levels are beyond your control. A psychotherapist can diagnose possible stress triggers and prescribe medications to aid in managing stress (Rockwell, 2011)

The Bible tells us that man born of woman is full of trouble (Job 14:1). Thus, God in His mercy offers help for those who are in trouble. Jesus invites us to come to Him with all of our troubles, anxieties, and problems (Matthew 11:28). He will give us rest. Turning to God should not be the last option, but the first. Many times we want to carry our own burdens, but Jesus calls us to bring all of our troubles to Him. We spend so much time worrying instead of praying. This is how our health is affected. Jesus continues to invite each of us to seek first His kingdom and His righteousness, and all other things will be given to us (Matthew 6:33), according to His best will for us. Look upon Jesus; He will see you through your troubles.

Psalms 23 tells us that the Lord is our Shepherd; He is the one who leads us into green pastures. He leads us beside the calm waters and restores our souls (giving us peace and easing our worries). He leads us in the right ways of life. Even though there may be troubles around, we should fear no evil, for Jesus is with us. Surely goodness and mercy shall follow us all the days of our lives and we shall dwell in the house of the Lord our whole lives (Psalms 23:6 NRSV).

We should dwell in the presence of God. Believe me or not, this is the best medicine for the heart and soul. In fact, this is the only way to be happy and live a healthy life. Jesus is the answer to your everyday problems. You will not regret giving him your life today. He waits to hear from you today. "I stand at the door knocking; if you hear my voice and open the door I will come in to you and with me" (Revelation 3:20 NRSV).

Conclusion

As one of my friends once said, "we should stop being attacked by anything in this world which perishes, but look to eternal Jesus all the time." Through your troubles, look to Jesus. He is the way and solution to our unresolved issues.

Let me conclude this chapter with a story I heard when I was about 15 years old. The story was about an old lady who was carrying heavy firewood on her head. A man with a truck passed by and saw this dear mother carrying firewood. He stopped and said, "Mother, please let me carry your firewood to your home." The old lady answered, "No, my son, just go on, I do not want to delay you from where you're going." The man insisted on helping her. She finally agreed and got into the back of the truck. However, she kept the firewood on her head. When the driver saw what was happening in the back of his truck, he stopped and said, "Mother, I carried you so you could rest from carrying your firewood. What is happening?" The lady said, "It is okay, my son, I did not want your truck to be heavy." She continued to carry it up to her destination. Unfortunately, when she got home, her neck was injured. The outcome was not good.

The message in this story is that when Jesus calls and offer to help us, we should accept it. If we refuse, the burden we're carrying in our lives may kill us. The best way is to give your problems to Jesus. He wants to help us in our troubles. "Come to me; let me help you," Jesus says.

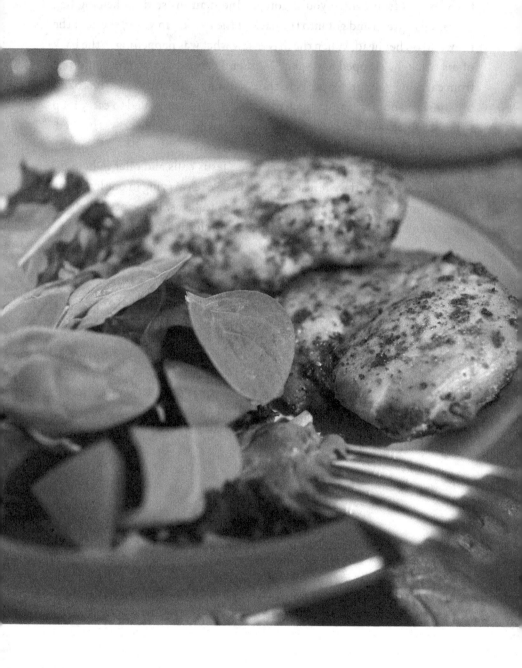

CHAPTER V

Aspects of Heart Disease

What Is Myocardial Infarction?

Myocardial infarction (MI) or acute myocardial infarction (AMI), commonly known as a heart attack, results from the partial interruption of blood supply to a part of the heart muscle, causing the heart cells to be damaged or die. This is most commonly due to occlusion (blockage) of a coronary artery following the rupture of a vulnerable atherosclerotic plaque, which is an unstable collection of cholesterol, fatty acids, and white blood cells in the wall of an artery (O'Connor, Brady, Brooks, 2010). The resulting ischemia (restriction in blood supply) and ensuing oxygen shortage, if left untreated for a sufficient period of time, can cause damage or death (infarction) of heart muscle tissue (myocardium).

Typical symptoms of acute myocardial infarction include sudden retrosternal chest pain (typically radiating to the left arm or left side of the neck), shortness of breath, nausea, vomiting, palpitations, sweating, and anxiety (often described as a sense of impending doom). Women may experience fewer typical symptoms than men, most commonly shortness of breath, weakness, a feeling of indigestion, and fatigue. A sizable proportion of myocardial infarctions (22–64%) are "silent," that is, without chest pain or other symptoms (Van de Werf, Bax, Betriu, 2008).

A number of diagnostic tests are available to detect heart muscle damage, including electrocardiograms (ECGs), echocardiography, cardiac MRI, and various blood tests. The most often used blood markers are the creatine kinase-MB (CK-MB) fraction and the troponin levels. Immediate treatment for suspected acute myocardial infarction includes oxygen, aspirin, and sublingual nitroglycerin.

Most cases of myocardial infarction with ST elevation on ECG (STEMI) are treated with reperfusion therapy, such as percutaneous coronary intervention (PCI) or thrombolysis. Non-ST elevation myocardial infarction (NSTEMI) may be managed with medication, although PCI may be required if the patient's risk warrants it. People who have multiple blockages of their coronary arteries, particularly if they also have diabetes mellitus, may benefit from bypass surgery (CABG) (Roe, Messenger, Weintraub, 2010).

The European Society of Cardiology guidelines in 2011 proposed treating the blockage causing the myocardial infarction by PCI and performing CABG later when the patient is more stable. Rarely CABG may be preferred in the acute phase of myocardial infarction, for example when PCI has failed or is contraindicated (Hamm, Bassand, Agewall, 2011)

Coronary Artery Disease

Coronary artery disease (CAD) is the leading cause of death in the United States, affecting over 5 million Americans. CAD is a narrowing of the coronary arteries, the vessels that supply blood to the heart muscle, generally due to the buildup of plaques in the arterial walls, a process known as atherosclerosis. Plaques are composed of cholesterol-rich fatty deposits, collagen, other proteins, and excess smooth muscle cells. Atherosclerosis, which usually progresses very gradually over a lifetime, thickens and narrows the arterial walls, impeding the flow of blood and starving the heart of the oxygen and vital nutrients it needs (also called "ischemia"). This can cause muscle cramp-like chest pain called angina.

Blood clots form more easily on arterial walls roughened by plaque deposits and may block one or more of the narrowed coronary arteries completely and cause a heart attack. Arteries may also narrow suddenly as a result of an arterial spasm (smoking commonly triggers spasms) (Berger, Buclin, Haller, Van Melle, Yersin, 1990).

Although CAD can be a life-threatening condition, the outcome of the disease is in many ways up to the patient. Damage to the arteries can be slowed or halted with lifestyle changes, including smoking cessation, dietary modifications, and regular exercise, or by medications to lower blood pressure and cholesterol levels. Additional goals of treatment, which may involve medication and sometimes surgery, are to relieve symptoms, ease circulation, and prolong life (Berger, Buclin, Haller, Van Melle, Yersin, 1990).

In the early stages of coronary artery disease, there are generally no symptoms, but the disease can start when a patient is very young (pre-teen). Over time, fat builds up and can injure the vessel walls where plaques will begin to adhere and collect. In an attempt to heal the troubled area, blood may form a clot around the plaque, causing the artery to narrow even further, preventing the flow of blood and oxygen, which can cause chest pain (angina pectoris) during periods of physical activity or emotional stress (times that require increased amounts of oxygen).

Angina usually subsides quickly with rest, but over time, symptoms arise with less exertion, and CAD may eventually lead to a heart attack. However, in one-third of all CAD cases, angina never develops and a heart attack can occur suddenly with no prior warning (Marcus, Cohen, Varosy, 2007).

Symptoms of coronary artery disease include the following:

- Chest pain (angina), or milder pressure, tightness, squeezing, burning, aching, or heaviness in the chest, lasting from 30 seconds to five minutes. The pain or discomfort is usually located in the center of the chest just under the breastbone and may radiate down the arm (usually the left), up into the neck or along the jawline. The pain is generally brought on by exertion or stress and stops with rest. The amount of exertion required to produce angina is reproducible and predictable. Angina can be mistaken for heartburn or indigestion.
- Shortness of breath, dizziness, or a choking sensation, accompanying chest pain.
- Rapid or irregular heartbeats.
- A sudden increase in the severity of angina, or angina at rest, is a sign of unstable angina that requires immediate medical attention because a heart attack may shortly occur (Canto, Goldberg, Hand, 2007)

In CAD, narrowed coronary arteries limit the supply of blood to the heart muscle. If narrowing is not extensive, difficulties may occur only during physical exertion, when the narrowed arteries are unable to meet the increased oxygen requirements of the heart. However, as the disease worsens, the narrowed arteries may starve the heart muscle of oxygen during periods of normal activity, or even at rest.

Lack of exercise may encourage atherosclerosis and lack of oxygenated blood circulation due to blockage of the arteries. Men are greater risk than women for coronary artery disease, although the risk for postmenopausal women approaches that of men as estrogen production decreases with menopause. Ongoing studies will determine whether this risk may be partly offset by estrogen replacement therapy (Davis, Fortun, Mulder, Davis, Bruce, 2004).

Ischemic heart disease (which includes myocardial infarction, angina pectoris, and heart failure when preceded by myocardial infarction) was the leading cause of death for both men and women worldwide in 2004.

Important risk factors are previous cardiovascular disease, older age, tobacco smoking, high blood levels of certain lipids (low-density lipoprotein cholesterol, triglycerides), low levels of high-density lipoprotein (HDL) cholesterol, diabetes, high blood pressure, lack of physical activity and obesity, chronic kidney disease, excessive alcohol consumption, the use of illicit drugs (such as cocaine and amphetamines), and chronic high stress levels.

There are two basic types of acute myocardial infarction based on pathology:

- Transmural: associated with atherosclerosis involving a major coronary artery. It can be subclassified into anterior, posterior, inferior, lateral, or septal. Transmural infarcts extend through the whole thickness of the heart muscle and are usually a result of complete occlusion of the area's blood supply. In addition, on ECG, ST elevation and Q waves are seen.
- Subendocardial: involving a small area in the subendocardial wall of the left ventricle, ventricular septum, or papillary muscles. The subendocardial area is particularly susceptible to ischemia. In addition, ST depression is seen on ECG (Buse, Ginsberg, Bakris, 2007).

The onset of symptoms in myocardial infarction is usually gradual, over several minutes, and rarely instantaneous. Chest pain is the most common symptom of acute myocardial infarction and is often described as a sensation of tightness, pressure, or squeezing (Nyboe, Jensen, Appleyard, Schnohr, 1989). Heart attack rates are higher in association with intense exertion, be it psychological stress or physical exertion, especially if the exertion is more intense than the individual usually performs.

The period of intense exercise and subsequent recovery is associated with about a sixfold higher myocardial infarction rate (compared with other more relaxed time frames) for people who are very physically fit. For those in poor physical condition, the rate differential is over 35-fold higher. One observed mechanism for this phenomenon is increased pulse pressure, which increases stretching of the arterial walls. This stretching results in significant shear stress on atheromas, which results in debris breaking loose from these deposits (Boie, 2005). This debris floats through the blood vessels, eventually clogging the major coronary arteries.

Acute severe infection, such as pneumonia, can also trigger myocardial infarction. A more controversial link is that between *Chlamydophila pneumoniae* infection and atherosclerosis. While this intracellular organism has been demonstrated in atherosclerotic plaques, evidence is inconclusive as to whether it can be considered a causative factor (Roe, Messenger, Weintraub, 2010).

Treatment with antibiotics in patients with proven atherosclerosis has not demonstrated a decreased risk of heart attacks or other coronary vascular diseases. There is an association with increased incidence of heart attack in the morning hours, more specifically around 9 a.m. Some investigators have noticed that the ability of platelets to aggregate varies according to a circadian rhythm, although they have not proven causation.

Conclusion

Smoking, drinking, eating an unhealthy diet, and stress are the main factors for heart disease. These habits can be avoided; they are not essential to survival. For those who are diabetic, it is best to avoid fats and high-cholesterol foods. Exercising and eating fruits and vegetable will lead to improvement in type 2 diabetes and will help to open the cell receptors.

Animal foods were never good for human consumption, and consuming animal products may not improve our health. When people eat anything which has eyes (animal flesh), they will suffer consequences. So many diseases exist because of eating and drinking habits; all these can be avoided.

Ellen G. White says in her book *Ministry of Healing*, "The diet appointed to man in the beginning did not include animal foods ... after the flood when every green thing on earth had been destroyed, man received permission to eat flesh." What was meant to be a temporary food has been made a permanent food for humans. No wonder we suffer with heart disease more than when the world was created. I have heard some people say they cannot go a day without eating meat. My point here is that whether you eat meat daily or once in a while, it is never good for you. If you keep eating it while knowing it is not good for you, someday you will pay a heavy penalty in health problems.

Remember, the Bible says that in times of ignorance (when you did not know) God pretended as if He did not see what you were doing, but since now you know, He will hold you accountable (Acts 17:30). God and science have shown us that meat was never good for us. Even modern medicine may not save us from contracting heart diseases through consumption of animal flesh.

People are worried about missing protein. The truth is that there are many sources of protein. Look at the cows and all other big herbivores; they eat no meat, yet see how big they become. They are strong and healthy, so you cannot claim protein from animal foods to be something you cannot live without.

"In choosing man's food in Eden, the Lord showed his people what was the best diet. In the choice he made for Israel, he brought the same lesson ... It was only because of their discontent and their murmuring for the fleshpots of Egypt that animal food was granted them and this only for a short time" (White, 2007).

These animal foods brought disease and death to thousands of them, yet they would rather die than live without animal flesh. God allowed them to have flesh meat because of their insistence. The word of God says, "While the meat was still in their teeth, they started dying." Hence, this reminds us not to eat anything with blood.

CHAPTER VI

Effects of Fats on the Heart

Fats from animal and vegetable sources provide a concentrated source of energy in the diet, they also provide the building blocks for cell membranes and a variety of hormones and hormone-like substances. Fats as part of a meal slow down absorption so that we can go longer without feeling hungry. In addition, they act as carriers for the important fat-soluble vitamins A, D, E, and K. Dietary fats are needed for the conversion of carotene to vitamin A, for mineral absorption, and for a host of other processes (Addis, 1990)

Animal Fats and Heart Disease

Fats from animals contain cholesterol, which may cause problems for the heart vessels. We should avoid animal fats.

The most well-known advocate of the low-fat diet was Nathan Pritikin. Pritikin advocated elimination of sugar, white flour, and all processed foods from the diet and recommended fresh raw foods, whole grains, and a strenuous exercise program; but it was the low-fat aspects of his regime that received the most attention in the media (Ahlen, 1998). Adherents found that they lost weight and that their cholesterol levels and blood pressure declined, but the success of the Pritikin diet was probably due to a number of factors having nothing to do with reduction in dietary fat. Those who possessed enough willpower to remain fat-free for any length of time developed a variety of health problems including low energy, difficulty in concentration, depression, weight gain, and mineral deficiencies (Gittleman, Louise, 1980).

Before 1920, coronary heart disease was rare in America; so rare that when a young internist named Paul Dudley White introduced the German electrocardiograph to his colleagues at Harvard University, they advised him to concentrate on a more profitable branch of medicine. The new machine revealed the presence of arterial blockages, permitting early diagnosis of coronary heart disease. But in those days clogged arteries were a medical rarity, and White had to search for patients who could benefit from his new technology. During the next 40 years, however, the incidence of coronary heart disease rose dramatically, so much so that by the mid-1950s heart disease was the leading cause of death among Americans (Hubert, 1983).

As stated before, heart disease causes at least 40% of all US deaths. We have been told that heart disease results from the consumption of saturated fats, so one would expect to find a corresponding increase in animal fat in the American diet. Actually, the reverse is true. During the 60-year period from 1910 to 1970, the proportion of traditional animal fat in the American diet declined from 83% to 62%, and butter consumption plummeted from 18 pounds per person per year to four. During the same period the percentage of dietary vegetable oils in the form of margarine, shortening, and refined oils increased about 400%, while the consumption of sugar and processed foods increased about 60% (Enig, 1995).

Classification of Fatty Acids

Fatty acids are classified in the following way:

Saturated

A fatty acid is saturated when all available carbon bonds are occupied by a hydrogen atom. They are highly stable, because all the carbon-atom linkages are filled—or saturated—with hydrogen. This means that they do not normally go rancid, even when heated for cooking purposes. They are straight in form and hence pack together easily, so that they form a solid or semisolid fat at room temperature. Your body makes saturated fatty acids from carbohydrates, and they are found in animal fats and tropical oils.

Monounsaturated

Monounsaturated fatty acids have one double bond in the form of two carbon atoms double-bonded to each other and, therefore, lack two hydrogen atoms. Your body makes monounsaturated fatty acids from saturated fatty acids and uses them in a number of ways. Monounsaturated fats have a kink or bend at the position of the double bond so that they do not pack together as easily as saturated fats and, therefore, tend to be liquid at room temperature. Like saturated fats, they are relatively stable. They do not go rancid easily and hence can be used in cooking. The monounsaturated fatty acid most commonly found in our food is oleic acid, the main component of olive oil as well as the oils from almonds, pecans, cashews, peanuts, and avocados.

Polyunsaturated

Polyunsaturated fatty acids have two or more pairs of double bonds and, therefore, lack four or more hydrogen atoms. The two polyunsaturated fatty acids found most frequently in our foods are double unsaturated linoleic acid, with two double bonds, also called omega-6, and triple unsaturated linoleic acid, with three double bonds, also called omega-3. (The omega number indicates the position of the first double bond.) Your body cannot make these fatty acids, and hence they are called "essential." We must obtain our essential fatty acids or EFA's from the foods we eat.

The polyunsaturated fatty acids have kinks or turns at the position of the double bond and hence do not pack together easily. They are liquid, even when refrigerated. The unpaired electrons at the double bonds make these oils highly reactive. They go rancid easily, particularly omega-3 linoleic acid, and must be treated with care. Polyunsaturated oils should never be heated or used in cooking. In nature, polyunsaturated fatty acids are usually found in the cis form, which means that both hydrogen atoms at the double bond are on the same side (Lovnskov, 1998).

All fats and oils, whether of vegetable or animal origin, are some combination of saturated fatty acids, monounsaturated fatty acids, and polyunsaturated linoleic acid and linoleic acid. In general, animal fats such as butter, lard, and tallow contain about 40-60% saturated fat and are solid at room temperature. Vegetable oils from northern climates contain a preponderance of polyunsaturated fatty acids and are liquid at room temperature. Vegetable oils from the tropics are highly saturated. Coconut oil, for example, is 92% saturated. These fats are liquid in the tropics, but hard as butter in northern climes. Vegetable oils are more saturated in hot climates because the increased saturation helps maintain stiffness in plant leaves. Olive oil with its preponderance of oleic acid is the product of a temperate climate. It is liquid at warm temperatures, but hardens when refrigerated (Holman, 1979).

Researchers classify fatty acids not only according to their degree of saturation but also by their length.

Short-Chain

Short-chain fatty acids have four to six carbon atoms. These fats are always saturated. Four-carbon butyric acid is found mostly in butterfat from cows, and six-carbon capric acid is found mostly in butterfat from goats. These fatty acids have antimicrobial properties—that is, they protect us from viruses, yeasts, and pathogenic bacteria in the gut. They do not need to be acted on by the bile salts, but are directly absorbed for quick energy. For this reason, they are less likely to cause weight gain than olive oil or commercial vegetable oils. Short-chain fatty acids also contribute to the health of the immune system (Kinsella, 1988).

Medium-Chain

Medium-chain fatty acids have eight to twelve carbon atoms and are found mostly in butterfat and the tropical oils. Like the short-chain fatty acids, these fats have antimicrobial properties, are absorbed directly for quick energy, and contribute to the health of the immune system.

Long-Chain

Long-chain fatty acids have 14 to 18 carbon atoms and can be either saturated, monounsaturated, or polyunsaturated. Stearic acid is an 18-carbon saturated fatty acid found chiefly in beef and mutton tallows. Oleic acid is an 18-carbon monounsaturated fat that is the chief component of olive oil.

Another monounsaturated fatty acid is the 16-carbon palmitoleic acid, which has strong antimicrobial properties. It is found almost exclusively in animal fats. The two essential fatty acids are also long-chain, each 18 carbons in length. Another important long-chain fatty acid is gamma-linoleic acid (GLA), which has 18 carbons and three double bonds. It is found in evening primrose, borage, and blackcurrant oils. Your body makes GLA out of omega-6 linoleic acid and uses it in the production of substances called prostaglandins, localized tissue hormones that regulate many processes at the cellular level.

Very-long-chain fatty acids have 20 to 24 carbon atoms. They tend to be highly unsaturated, with four, five, or six double bonds. Some people can make these fatty acids from EFAs, but others, particularly those whose ancestors ate a lot of fish, lack enzymes to produce them. These "obligate carnivores" must obtain them from animal foods such as organ meats, egg yolks, butter, and fish oils (Lackland, 1990). The most important very-long-chain fatty acids are dihomo-gamma-linoleic acid (DGLA) with 20 carbons and three double bonds; arachidonic acid (AA) with 20 carbons and four double bonds; eicosapentaenoic acid (EPA) with 20 carbons and five double bonds; and docosahexaenoic acid (DHA) with 22 carbons and six double bonds. All of these except DHA are used in the production of prostaglandins. In addition, AA and DHA play important roles in the function of the nervous system (Horrobin, 1983).

The Dangers of Polyunsaturated Oils

The public has been fed a great deal of misinformation about the relative virtues of saturated fats versus polyunsaturated oils. Politically correct dietary gurus tell us that the polyunsaturated oils are good for us and that the saturated fats cause cancer and heart disease. The result is that fundamental changes have occurred in the Western diet. At the turn of the century, most of the fatty acids in the diet were either saturated or monounsaturated, primarily from butter, lard, tallow, coconut oil, and small amounts of olive oil. Today, most of the fats in the diet are polyunsaturated from vegetable oils derived mostly from soy, as well as from corn, safflower, and canola.

Modern diets can contain as much as 30% of calories as polyunsaturated oils, but scientific research indicates that this amount is far too high. The best evidence indicates that our intake of polyunsaturated oils should not be much greater than 4% of the caloric total, in approximate proportions of 1 1/2 % omega-3 linoleic acid and 2 1/2 % omega-6 linoleic acid (Okuyama, 1997). EFA consumption in this range is found in native populations in temperate and tropical regions whose intake of polyunsaturated oils comes from the small amounts found in legumes, grains, nuts, green vegetables, fish, olive oil, and animal fats, but not from commercial vegetable oils. Excess consumption of polyunsaturated oils has been shown to contribute to a large number of disease conditions including increased cancer and heart disease; immune system dysfunction; damage to the liver, reproductive organs, and lungs; digestive disorders; depressed learning ability; impaired growth; and weight gain (Edward, Pinckney, 1990).

One reason the polyunsaturated oils cause so many health problems is that they tend to become oxidized or rancid when subjected to heat, oxygen, and moisture, as in cooking and processing. Rancid oils are characterized by free radicals—that is, single atoms or clusters with an unpaired electron in an outer orbit. These compounds are extremely reactive chemically. They have been characterized as "marauders" in the body, for they attack cell membranes and red blood cells and cause damage in DNA/RNA strands, thus triggering mutations in tissue, blood vessels, and skin. Free radical damage to the skin causes wrinkles and premature aging; free radical damage to the tissues and organs sets the stage for tumors; free radical damage in the blood vessels initiates the buildup of plaque. Is it any wonder that tests and studies have repeatedly shown a high correlation between cancer and heart disease and the consumption of polyunsaturated oils? New evidence links exposure to free radicals with premature aging, autoimmune disease (Watkins, 1996) such as arthritis, Parkinson's disease, Lou Gehrig's disease, Alzheimer's, and cataracts.

Too Much Omega-6

Problems associated with an excess of polyunsaturates are exacerbated by the fact that most polyunsaturates in commercial vegetable oils are in the form of double unsaturated omega-6 linoleic acid, with very little of vital triple unsaturated omega-3 linoleic acid. Recent research has revealed that too much omega-6 in the diet creates an imbalance that can interfere with production of important prostaglandins (Pinckney, Edward, Pinckney, 1978).

This disruption can result in increased tendency to form blood clots, inflammation, high blood pressure, irritation of the digestive tract, depressed immune function, sterility, cell proliferation, cancer, and weight gain (Pinckney, Edward, Pinckney, 1978).

Too Little Omega-3

A number of researchers have argued that along with a surfeit of omega-6 fatty acids, the American diet is deficient in the more unsaturated omega-3 linoleic acid. This fatty acid is necessary for cell oxidation, for metabolizing important sulfur-containing amino acids, and for maintaining proper balance in prostaglandin production. Deficiencies have been associated with asthma, heart disease, and learning deficiencies (Fallon, Sally, Enig, 1996).

Most commercial vegetable oils contain very little omega-3 linoleic acid and large amounts of omega-6 linoleic acid. In addition, modern agricultural and industrial practices have reduced the amount of omega-3 fatty acids in commercially available vegetables, eggs, fish, and meat. For example, organic eggs from hens allowed to feed on insects and green plants can contain omega-6 and omega-3 fatty acids in the beneficial ratio of approximately one-to-one, but commercial supermarket eggs can contain as much as 19 times more omega-6 than omega-3 (Fallon, Sally, Enig, 1996).

The Benefits of Saturated Fats

The much-maligned saturated fats—which Americans are trying to avoid— are not the cause of our modern diseases. In fact, they play many important roles in the body chemistry:

- Saturated fatty acids constitute at least 50% of the cell membranes. They are what give our cells necessary stiffness and integrity.
- They play a vital role in the health of our bones. For calcium to be effectively incorporated into the skeletal structure, at least 50% of the dietary fats should be saturated.

- They lower substances in the blood that indicate proneness to heart disease. They protect the liver from alcohol and other toxins, such as Tylenol.
- They enhance the immune system.
- They are needed for the proper utilization of essential fatty acids. Elongated omega-3 fatty acids are better retained in the tissues when the diet is rich in saturated fats.
- Saturated 18-carbon stearic acid and 16-carbon palmitic acid are the preferred foods for the heart, which is why the fat around the heart muscle is highly saturated. The heart draws on this reserve of fat in times of stress (Lawson, 1979).
- Short- and medium-chain saturated fatty acids have important antimicrobial properties. They protect us against harmful microorganisms in the digestive tract.

Our blood vessels can become damaged in a number of ways—through irritations caused by free radicals or viruses, or because they are structurally weak—and when this happens, the body's natural healing substance steps in to repair the damage. The cholesterol substance is a high-molecular-weight alcohol that is manufactured in the liver and in most human cells, like saturated fats.

When the diet contains an excess of polyunsaturated fatty acids, these replace saturated fatty acids in the cell membrane, so that the cell walls actually become flabby. When this happens, the blood cholesterol is "driven" into the tissues to give them structural integrity. This is why serum level of cholesterol may go down temporarily when we replace saturated fats with polyunsaturated oils in the diet.

Cholesterol acts as a precursor to vital corticosteroids (hormones that help us deal with stress and protect the body against heart disease and cancer) and sex hormones like androgen, testosterone, estrogen, and progesterone.

Cholesterol is a precursor to vitamin D, a very important fat-soluble vitamin needed for healthy bones and nervous system, proper growth, mineral metabolism, muscle tone, insulin production, reproduction, and immune system function.

The bile salts are made from cholesterol; bile is vital for digestion and assimilation of fats in the diet.

Oil Extraction

Oils naturally occurring in fruits, nuts, and seeds must first be extracted. In the old days, slow-moving stone presses achieved this extraction. But crushing the oil-bearing seeds and heating them to 230 degrees is how oils are processed in large factories. The oil is then squeezed out at pressures from 10 to 20 tons per inch, thereby generating more heat. During this process, the oils are exposed to damaging light and oxygen. In order to extract the last 10% or so of the oil from crushed seeds, processors treat the pulp with one of a number of solvents—usually hexane. The solvent is then boiled off, although up to 100 parts per million may remain in the oil. Such solvents, themselves toxic, also retain the toxic pesticides adhering to seeds and grains before processing begins.

High-temperature processing causes the weak carbon bonds of unsaturated fatty acids, especially triple unsaturated linoleic acid, to break apart, thereby creating dangerous free radicals. In addition, antioxidants, such as fat-soluble vitamin E, which protect the body from the ravages of free radicals, are neutralized or destroyed by high temperatures and pressures (Alfin-Slater, Aftergood, 1980).

Expeller-expressed, unrefined oils will remain fresh for a long time if stored in the refrigerator in dark bottles. Crushing olives between stone or steel rollers produces extra virgin olive oil. This process is a gentle one that preserves the integrity of the fatty acids and the numerous natural preservatives in olive oil. If olive oil is packaged in opaque containers, it will retain its freshness and precious store of antioxidants for many years.

Hydrogenation and Homogenization

Hydrogenation is the process that turns polyunsaturates, normally liquid at room temperature, into fats that are solid at room temperature—margarine and shortening. To produce them, manufacturers begin with the cheapest oils—soy, corn, cottonseed, or canola, already rancid from the extraction process—and mix them with tiny metal particles—usually nickel oxide. The oil with its nickel catalyst is then subjected to hydrogen gas in a high-pressure, high-temperature reactor. Next, soap-like emulsifiers and starch are squeezed into the mixture to give it a better consistency; the oil is yet again subjected to high temperatures when it is steam-cleaned. This removes its unpleasant odor. Margarine's natural color, an unappetizing grey, is removed by bleach. Dyes and strong flavors must then be added to make it resemble butter.

Finally, the mixture is compressed and packaged in blocks or tubs and sold as a health food. Partially hydrogenated margarines and shortenings are even worse for you than the highly refined vegetable oils from which they are made because of chemical changes that occur during the hydrogenation process. Under high temperatures, the nickel catalyst causes the hydrogen atoms to change position on the fatty acid chain. Before hydrogenation, pairs of hydrogen atoms occur together on the chain, causing the chain to bend slightly and creating a concentration of electrons at the site of the double bond. This is called the cis formation, the configuration most commonly found in nature. With hydrogenation, one hydrogen atom of the pair is moved to the other side so that the molecule straightens. This is called the trans formation, rarely found in nature. Most of these man-made trans fats are toxins to the body, but unfortunately your digestive system does not recognize them as such. Instead of being eliminated, trans fats are incorporated into cell membranes as if they were cis fats—your cells actually become partially hydrogenated! Once in place, trans fatty acids with their misplaced hydrogen atoms wreak havoc in cell metabolism because chemical reactions can only take place when electrons in the cell membranes are in certain arrangements or patterns, which the hydrogenation process has disturbed (Enig, 1995).

Natural saturated fats have been tarred with the black brush of unnatural hydrogenated vegetable oils. Altered partially hydrogenated fats made from vegetable oils actually block utilization of essential fatty acids, causing many deleterious effects including sexual dysfunction, increased cholesterol in the blood, and paralysis of the immune system. Consumption of hydrogenated fats is associated with a host of other serious diseases: not only cancer but also atherosclerosis, diabetes, obesity, immune system dysfunction, low-birth-weight babies, birth defects, decreased visual acuity, sterility, difficulty in lactation, and problems with bones and tendons (Alfin-Slater, Aftergood, 1980).

Yet hydrogenated fats continue to be promoted as health foods. The popularity of partially hydrogenated margarine over butter represents a triumph of advertising duplicity over common sense. Your best defense is to avoid it like the plague.

Homogenization is the process whereby the fat particles of cream are strained through tiny pores under great pressure. The resulting fat particles are so small that they stay in suspension rather than rise to the top of the milk. This makes the fat more susceptible to rancidity and oxidation, and some research indicates that homogenized fats may contribute to heart disease (Engelberg, 1992).

Fat-Soluble Vitamins and Other Possible Benefits of Butterfat

Fat-soluble vitamins include true vitamin A or retinol, vitamin D, vitamin K, and vitamin E, as well as all their naturally occurring cofactors needed to obtain maximum effect. Vitamins A and D are essential for growth, for healthy bones, for proper development of the brain and nervous systems, and for normal sexual development (Alfin-Slater, Aftergood 1980)

Lecithin is a natural component of butter that assists in the proper assimilation and metabolization of cholesterol and other fat constituents.

Mother's milk is high in cholesterol because it is essential for growth and development Cholesterol is also needed to produce a variety of steroids that protect against cancer, heart disease, and mental illness.

Glycosphingolipids protect against gastrointestinal infections, especially in the very young and the elderly. For this reason, children who drink skimmed milk have diarrhea at rates three to five times greater than children who drink whole milk (Smith, Lifshitz, 1994)

Many trace minerals are incorporated into the fat globule membrane of butterfat, including manganese, zinc, chromium, and iodine. In mountainous areas far from the sea, iodine in butter protects against goiter. Butter is extremely rich in selenium, a trace mineral with antioxidant properties, containing more per gram than herring or wheat germ.

One frequently voiced objection to the consumption of butter and other animal fats is that they tend to accumulate environmental poisons. However, the solution to environmental poisons is not to eliminate animal fats—so essential to growth, reproduction and overall health—but to seek out organic meats and butter from pasture-fed cows, as well as organic vegetables and grains (Watson, 1996).

Composition of Different Fats

Before leaving this complex but vital subject of fats, it is worthwhile examining the composition of vegetable oils and other animal fats in order to determine their usefulness and appropriateness in food preparation.

Olive Oil

Olive oil contains 75% oleic acid, the stable monounsaturated fat, along with 13% saturated fat, 10% omega-6 linoleic acid, and 2% omega-3 linoleic acid. The high percentage of oleic acid makes olive oil ideal for salads and for cooking at moderate temperatures.

Extra virgin olive oil is also rich in antioxidants. It should be cloudy, indicating that it has not been filtered, and have a golden yellow color, indicating that it is made from fully ripened olives. Olive oil has withstood the test of time; it is the safest vegetable oil you can use, but don't overdo. The longer-chain fatty acids found in olive oil are more likely to contribute to the buildup of body fat than the short- and medium-chain fatty acids found in butter, coconut oil, or palm kernel oil.

Peanut Oil

Peanut oil contains 48% oleic acid, 18% saturated fat, and 34% omega-6 linoleic acid. Like olive oil, peanut oil is relatively stable and, therefore, appropriate for stir-frying on occasion. But the high percentage of omega-6 presents a potential danger, so use of peanut oil should be strictly limited.

Sesame Oil

Sesame oil contains 42% oleic acid, 15% saturated fat, and 43% omega-6 linoleic acid. Sesame oil is similar in composition to peanut oil. It can be used for frying because it contains unique antioxidants that are not destroyed by heat. However, the high percentage of omega-6 militates against exclusive use.

Safflower, Corn, Sunflower, Soybean, and Cottonseed Oils.

These all contain over 50% omega-6 and, except for soybean oil, only minimal amounts of omega-3. Safflower oil contains almost 80% omega-6. Researchers are just beginning to discover the dangers of excess omega-6 oils in the diet, whether rancid or not. Use of these oils should be strictly limited. They should never be consumed after they have been heated, as in cooking, frying, or baking.

High-oleic safflower and sunflower oils, produced from hybrid plants, have a composition similar to olive oil, namely, high amounts of oleic acid and only small amounts of polyunsaturated fatty acids; thus, they are more stable than traditional varieties. However, it is difficult to find truly cold-pressed versions of these oils.

Canola Oil

Canola oil ontains 5% saturated fat, 57% oleic acid, 23% omega-6, and 10%-15% omega-3. The newest oil on the market, canola oil was developed from the rapeseed, a member of the mustard family. Rapeseed is unsuited to human consumption because it contains a very-long-chain fatty acid called erucic acid, which under some circumstances is associated with fibrotic heart lesions. Canola oil was bred to contain little if any erucic acid and has drawn the attention of nutritionists because of its high oleic acid content. But there are some indications that canola oil presents dangers of its own.

Flax Seed Oil

Flax seed oil contains 9% saturated fatty acids, 18% oleic acid, 16% omega-6, and 57% omega-3. With its extremely high omega-3 content, flax seed oil provides a remedy for the omega-6/omega-3 imbalance so prevalent in America today. Not surprisingly, Scandinavian folklore values flax seed oil as a health food. New extraction and bottling methods have minimized rancidity problems. It should always be kept refrigerated, never heated, and consumed in small amounts in salad dressings and spreads (Fallon, Sally, Enig, 1996).

Tropical Oils

These are more saturated than other vegetable oils.

- **Palm oil** is about 50% saturated, with 41% oleic acid and about 9% linoleic acid. Even though palm oil is from a tree, it is not the best oil because at room temperature it gets hard. It will do the same in your heart vessels.
- **Coconut oil** is 92% saturated with over two-thirds of the saturated fat in the form of medium-chain fatty acids (often called medium-chain triglycerides). Of particular interest is lauric acid, found in large quantities in both coconut oil and in mother's milk. This fatty acid has strong antifungal and antimicrobial properties. Coconut oil protects tropical populations from bacteria and fungus so prevalent in their food supply; as third-world nations in tropical areas have switched to polyunsaturated vegetable oils, the incidence of intestinal disorders and immune deficiency diseases has increased dramatically. Because coconut oil contains lauric acid, it is often used in baby formulas.
- **Palm kernel oil**, used primarily in candy coatings, also contains high levels of lauric acid. These oils are extremely stable and can be kept at room temperature for many months without becoming rancid. Highly saturated tropical oils do not contribute to heart disease but have nourished healthy populations for millennia. It is a shame we do not use these oils for cooking and baking—the bad rap they have received is the result of intense lobbying by the domestic vegetable oil industry.
- **Red palm oil** has a strong taste that most will find disagreeable—although it is used extensively throughout Africa—but **clarified palm oil**, which is tasteless and white in color, was formerly used as shortening and in the production of commercial French fries, while coconut oil was used in cookies, crackers, and pastries.

The saturated fat scare has forced manufacturers to abandon these safe and healthy oils in favor of hydrogenated soybean, corn, canola, and cottonseed oils (Engelberg, 1992).

Conclusion

It must be clear in your mind that not all cholesterol is bad for your body. You need cholesterol for energy and for the proper function of your body. To be safe, plant oil is good, while animal fats are dangerous for your heart. You also need fat-soluble vitamins to maintain health, but they can be derived from plants, not from animal foods.

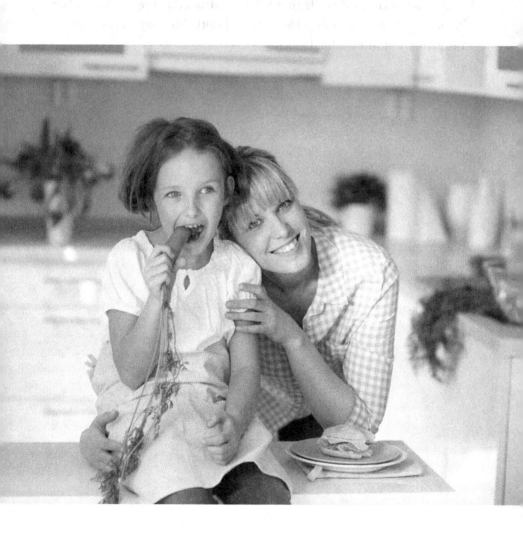

CHAPTER VII
Importance of Vitamins and Minerals

Vitamins

Vitamin A

Vitamin A is known to help with vision and skin maintenance. Without it, vision and cell division do not work well. This vitamin is important in the rod and cone cells of the eyes. It helps with hair growth and night vision, and prevents blindness. It is also known for balancing hypothyroid hormone.

Too much vitamin A may cause hyperthyroidism; too little can cause calcium to be low and then cause hypothyroidism. Excess vitamin A can cause the symptoms of pancreatitis or a pseudotumor of the cerebrum, which presents with headache and papilledema, heart ventricle enlargement, and high blood pressure.

Vitamin B1 (Thiamine)

This vitamin is also called pyruvate dehydrogenase. It has alfa keto glutarate dehydrogenase and branched chain amino acid dehydrogenase as well as transketolase, which affects the left temporal lobe and cures the effects of alcohol impairment by working on Wernicke and Korsakoff in the mammillary bodies (triggers confabulation and psychosis due to alcohol use).

Vitamin B1 deficiencies are called wet beriberi (high output cardiac failure) and dry beriberi (no heart failure).

Vitamin B2 (Riboflavin, FADH2)

A lack of vitamin B2 can cause angular cheliosis, which means wounds on the corners of your mouth. It may also cause stomatitis, in which the body starts breaking down and you get unexplained wounds on your skin.

Vitamin B2 can be found in milk and vegetables. I remember working in Africa for six months without eating vegetables or drinking milk. My body started breaking down in ways that I could not understand. Some of my best friends asked me what was happening, and I said it was because I was not eating right. After I returned to the U.S. and started eating right, my body recovered. It takes about six months for the body to break down if it does not get the nutrients it needs.

The sun can break down this vitamin, which is why milk is no longer stored in glass bottles.

Vitamin B3 (Niacin)

This vitamin helps people with high cholesterol. It is also called NAD/NADH.

Niacin deficiency will cause pellagra, which involves the three Ds (dementia, diarrhea, dermatitis) and can cause death if not treated. Hartnup's disease or defective renal transport presents very similarly, and may affect the heart.

Tryptophan is needed to make niacin. Niacin is what makes omega-3 from seeds and fish, as mentioned before in this book.

Vitamin B6 (Pyridoxine)

This vitamin is also used to treat people with tuberculosis.

It is a cofactor for all transaminases. A deficiency of this vitamin will cause neuropathy (a mental problem).

Vitamin B9 (Folate)

This is the first vitamin to run out in association with rapidly dividing cells and is found in raw vegetables. It only takes about six months to be depleted from the body. If folate is depleted in the body, it may cause the same symptoms as B2 deficiency.

Deficiencies of this vitamin during pregnancy can cause neural tube defects in the fetus (the spinal cord is not formed correctly).

Vitamin B12 (Cyanocobalamin)

This vitamin is essential for children's growth. It is mainly found in animal products. It is a methyl malonyl CoA mutase and is needed in prevention of myelin neuropathy (works with brain functions). The vitamin is water-soluble, although absorbed in proximal ileum.

- Deficiency of this vitamin will cause deformity of the dorsal column/cortical spinal tracts because they are the longest tracts.
- Deficiency of this vitamin may also cause megaloblastic anemia, meaning the cells become big and fail to divide.

Children need vitamin B12 for forming the spinal cord and growth, and they must have enough of it from conception.

Adults do not need as much. In adults, this vitamin stays in the body for 12 months. So, if you eat animal products for B12 once a year, you will be good to go if you do not have diabetes or consume alcohol.

Vitamin C

This vitamin is found in fruits. Vitamin C deficiency is called scurvy, and causes bleeding gums and hair follicles. This vitamin is needed for collagen synthesis (bending and flexibility), catecholamine synthesis (a neurotransmitter hormone), and absorption of iron in the GI tract. It also helps remove free radicals. It is imperative to eat fruits daily to reduce free radicals in the body.

Vitamin D

This vitamin helps maintain our bones and teeth. It is involved in calcium absorption in the gut and reabsorption of calcium from the kidneys. It aids in osteoplastic activity by increasing levels of both calcium and potassium.

Vitamin D deficiency may cause rickets (a lateral bowing of legs) and osteomalacia (soft bones).

Vitamin E

This vitamin comes from green foods. It is an antioxidant (absorbs free radicals). It is good for the skin, eyes, and hair. Women who buy topical vitamin E products for their hair should be aware that eating vegetables rich in the vitamin is better for hair growth.

Vitamin E deficiency may trigger retinopathy (a vision problem) and Alzheimer's (in elders and Down syndrome patients).

Vitamin H

- Clotting factors 2, 7, 9, 10, (1972), proteins C (shortest half-life) and S.
- γ-carboxylation of these factors.

Minerals

Iron (Fe2+)

Iron is an essential part of hemoglobin, which transports oxygen in the blood. It also supports the electron transport chain complexes III/IV. Iron deficiency can cause possible mental retardation in children.

Calcium (Ca2+)

Calcium is necessary for muscle contraction, including the heart muscle. Without it, the heart will have a hard time contracting. All muscles need intracellular calcium; cardiac and smooth muscles also need extracellular calcium for atrial contraction, also called the IP3/DAG second messenger system.

Magnesium (Mg2+)

This is a cofactor for all kinases and PTH.

Copper (Cu2+)

Copper is needed for the hydroxylation of lysine. A copper deficiency will produce Minky's kinky hair—orange hair that feels like copper wiring. Too much copper will cause Wilson's disease or hepatolenticular degeneration.

Zinc (Zn)

This mineral affects the hair, taste buds, and sperm production. A lack of it may cause one to lose the sense of taste and produce less sperm. This is mostly common in elderly people and people in a low-energy state (including diabetics).

Chromium

This mineral is needed for the action of insulin as well as for heart function.

Conclusion

Vitamins and minerals are necessary to maintain our body function and remain healthy. Please bear in mind that a bad lifestyle destroys their function quickly. For example, tobacco use destroys the taste buds and zinc. For better health, take care of yourself.

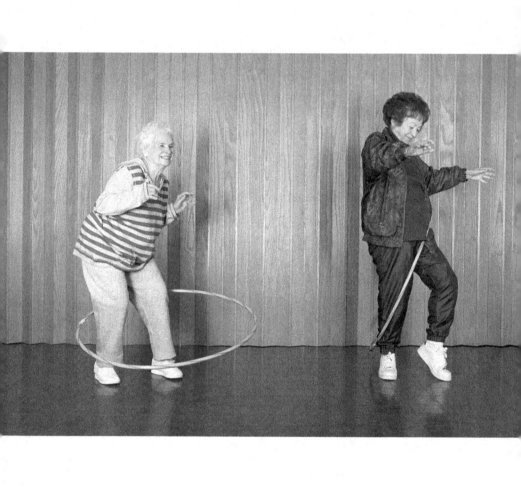

CHAPTER VIII

The Effects of Medicine

This chapter will help you understand the effects of some common medicines. It will also help you to see the good and bad of taking medicine. The goal is to help you take care of your health as well as understand the risk of taking medication for your survival.

I am not suggesting you should not take medicine when you're sick. However, the emphasis is on keeping yourself from getting sick through preventive methods.

I was born in Tanzania, where I did not have many foods. When I went to Sweden and the United States, I started eating like Swedish and American people. Before I knew it, I had gained weight and started losing energy. When checked by a physician, I was diagnosed with type 2 diabetes. I took medicine for more than five years. It did not change my situation.

I took the medication to help me with my diabetes, but nothing worked out. When I changed my lifestyle to eat unrefined foods and exercise, my health came back to me. I do not take medicine. I am always reminded when I eat unhealthy foods.

Let us now look to common medications and how they help and affect us.

Aspirin

Aspirin can prevent blood clot formations that block the coronary arteries and cause heart attacks. Research in patients with unstable angina has proven that taking an aspirin every day reduces the risk of heart attack. Acetaminophen (Tylenol) and ibuprofen (Advil) are not the same as aspirin, and should not be used in place of aspirin .Use these drugs only when necessary. There are some natural foods like walnuts and garlic that can do the same thing with fewer side effects (Hamm, Bassand, Agewall, 2011).

If your have unstable angina, you will probably be told to take aspirin every day. If you are dependent on such a protocol, I am not saying you should stop taking medication, but you should work with your physician to find the cause of your problem. Then you can consider changing your lifestyle. When you do so, you will see changes in your life. Maybe you will eventually stop taking medications altogether after checking with your primary care doctor, depending on how conservative you are with your new lifestyle.

I am not suggesting stopping your medication without checking with your physician. An early checkup will determine how you're doing with your health and lifestyle. However, the truth is that changing your lifestyle may work better than pharmaceutical treatments. There are foods that, if used properly, may work the same way aspirin works, such as garlic and some nuts.

ACE Inhibitors

ACE inhibitors—including captopril, enalapril, lisinopril, and quinapril—help to keep blood vessels from narrowing. They lower blood pressure and keep the heart from working too hard to pump blood. ACE inhibitors have been shown to help heart failure patients live longer and feel better, but it may take a few weeks before they feel better from taking the medicine.

Possible side effects of ACE inhibitors include:

- Coughing
- Dizziness
- Skin rash
- Fluid retention
- Excess potassium in the bloodstream
- Kidney problems
- Altered or lost sense of taste

Beta-Blockers

Beta-blockers can decrease the amount of work the heart needs to do and the amount of oxygen it needs.

Possible side effects of beta-blockers include:

- Dizziness
- Fatigue
- Depression
- Diarrhea
- Skin rash
- Mental confusion
- Headaches
- Heartburn
- Shortness of breath (Heidenreich, Trogdon, Khavjou, 2011)

Calcium-Channel Blockers

Calcium-channel blockers relax blood vessels and treat high blood pressure and chest pain.

Possible side effects of calcium-channel blockers include:

- Headaches
- Dizziness
- Nausea
- Bradycardia (slow heartbeat)
- Edema
- Asthenia (weakness)

Digitalis

Digitalis strengthens each heartbeat, allowing the heart to pump more blood. This may improve one's ability to exercise. Prescribed as digoxin or Lanoxin, digitalis is taken daily by many heart patients (Kannel, 1986).

Possible side effects of digitalis include:

- Nausea
- Loss of appetite
- Diarrhea
- Mental confusion

- Blurred or yellow-colored vision
- Rapid, forceful heartbeat (palpitations)

Diuretics

During physical activity, check with a physician about the effects of diuretics. The symptoms may also occur if doses are skipped.

The most commonly used diuretics are hydrochlorothiazide and furosemide (Lasix). Regular use of some diuretics can lead to the loss of potassium and to other nutritional imbalances. Blood tests are needed to monitor these levels. To replace lost potassium, you may have to do the following:

- Eat more foods rich in potassium (such as bananas and raisins)
- Drink orange juice and other citrus juices
- Take a prescribed potassium supplement

Possible side effects of diuretics include:

- Leg cramps
- Dizziness or lightheadedness
- Incontinence (accidental urine leakage)
- Gout (a type of arthritis)
- Skin rash
- Note: urinating more often is not a side effect; it is the intended result of the diuretic (Heidenreich, Trogdon, Khavjou, 2011)

Hydralazine

This drug widens blood vessels, easing blood flow.
Possible side effects of hydralazine include:

- Headaches
- Rapid heartbeat
- Joint pain

Insulin

The pancreas normally secretes a hormone called insulin, which helps move glucose from the blood into the body's cells. Cells in turn use glucose for energy. When functioning, as it should, the pancreas produces the ideal amount of insulin. In people with type 1 diabetes, the pancreas doesn't produce insulin. People with type 2 diabetes produce insulin, but their bodies do not use it properly. Over time with type 2 diabetes, less insulin is produced. Insulin may be prescribed for both types of diabetes to help regulate blood glucose so the body can work properly.

There are many types of insulin on the market, all of which must be injected into the fat under the skin in order for it to reach the bloodstream. (Insulin is not available in pill form because it would be broken down during the digestive process.) Injections can be done in several ways:

- **Syringe:** A needle connected to a hollow tube that holds the insulin and a plunger that pushes the insulin down into and through the needle
- **Insulin pen:** A device that looks like a pen and holds insulin but has a needle for its tip
- **Insulin pump:** A small machine (worn on a belt or kept in a pocket) that holds insulin, pumps it through a small plastic tube and through a tiny needle inserted under the skin where it stays for several days

Insulin types differ by how they are made, how quickly they work, when they peak, how long they last, and how much they cost. They include:

- **Rapid-acting insulin,** which begins to work about five minutes after injection, peaks about an hour later, and continues to work for two to four hours
- **Regular or short-acting insulin,** which usually gets into the bloodstream within 30 minutes of injection, peaks two to three hours after injection, and is effective for about three to six hours
- **Intermediate-acting insulin,** which typically gets into the bloodstream two to four hours after injection, peaks four to 12 hours later, and works for around 12 to 18 hours

- **Long-acting insulin**, which gets into the bloodstream six to ten hours after injection and remains effective for about 20 to 24 hours

Your doctor will work with you to determine the best type and dosage to manage your diabetes. Some patients take insulin one to four times a day to regulate their blood glucose levels. Your health care team may educate you about how and when to give yourself insulin. The side effects of insulin include low blood glucose and weight gain (Roge, Lloyd-Jones, 2012).

Nitrates

Nitrates (usually nitroglycerin and isosorbide) increase blood flow to the heart muscle and make it easier for the heart to work. They can relieve most angina discomfort very quickly. Nitrates are taken as tablets placed under the tongue, tablets that are swallowed, a patch worn on the skin, or a cream applied to the skin. Nitrate tablets, creams, and patches all have a limited shelf life; ask your pharmacist to explain the expiration dates. Nitrate creams and patches are for maintenance therapy only.

It is recommended that you should take one nitroglycerin tablet as soon as you feel any angina discomfort, or chest pain. If the discomfort does not go away in five minutes, take a second tablet. If it does not go away after five more minutes, take a third tablet. If the discomfort has not gone away after taking three nitrate tablets in 15 minutes, you should go to the hospital immediately. Persistent discomfort that doesn't go away could be a sign of a heart attack (Kannel, 1986).

While making lifestyle changes can go a long way in managing diabetes, as well as related conditions such as high blood pressure and high cholesterol, your doctor may prescribe medications depending on your health needs.

Your diabetes treatment plan may include insulin, oral diabetes medication, or a combination approach, as determined by your doctor. In some cases, patients may require multiple-drug therapy if they have additional cardiovascular risk factors with diabetes. Adherence to your medication plan is very important (Roger, Lloyd-Jones, 2012).

Oral Diabetic Medication

For people with type 2 diabetes or gestational diabetes (diabetes that develops during pregnancy), pills may be prescribed to regulate blood glucose levels. There are ten classes of oral diabetes medications that lower blood glucose. They can be used with insulin or in combination with one another. Your health care provider will prescribe the type of medication or combination of medications that you will need to lower your blood glucose levels (Buse, Ginsberg, Bakris, 2007).

Cholesterol Medication

Sometimes cholesterol medication is recommended in addition to a low-saturated-fat, low-refined-carbohydrate, and high-fiber diet to lower cholesterol.

Cholesterol is an important part of your cells and also serves as the building block of some hormones. The liver makes all the cholesterol the body needs. But cholesterol also enters your body from dietary sources, such as animal-based foods like milk, eggs, and meat.

Too much cholesterol in your blood can increase the risk of coronary artery disease even though moderate-cholesterol foods may be good for you.

For millions of people at risk for atherosclerosis complications, lifestyle changes aren't enough. Fortunately, medications are available to protect against atherosclerosis, or even partially reverse it.

The first line of treatment for abnormal cholesterol is usually to eat a diet low in saturated and trans fats, and high in fruits and vegetables, nuts, and seeds, and to increase exercise. But for some, these changes alone are not enough to lower blood cholesterol levels. These people may need medicine to bring their cholesterol down to a safe level.

Cholesterol-lowering drugs include:

- Statins
- Niacin
- Bile-acid resins
- Fibric acid derivatives
- Cholesterol absorption inhibitors

Cholesterol-lowering medicine is most effective when combined with a healthy diet and exercise.

Statins block the production of cholesterol in the liver itself. They lower LDL, the "bad" cholesterol, and triglycerides, and have a mild effect on raising HDL, the "good" cholesterol. These drugs are the first line of treatment for most people with high cholesterol.

Statins have been shown in multiple research studies to reduce the risk of cardiovascular events like heart attacks and death from heart disease. Side effects can include intestinal problems, liver damage, and in a few people, muscle tenderness.

Statins also carry warnings that memory loss, mental confusion, high blood sugar, and type 2 diabetes are possible side effects. It's important to remember that statins may also interact with other medications you take.

Examples of statins include:

- Atorvastatin (Lipitor)
- Fluvastatin (Lescol)
- Lovastatin (Mevacor)
- Pravastatin (Pravachol)
- Simvastatin (Zocor)
- Rosuvastatin (Crestor)

Nicotinic acid or niacin is a B-complex vitamin. It's found in food, but is also available at high doses by prescription. It lowers LDL cholesterol and raises HDL cholesterol. The main side effects are flushing, itching, tingling, and headache. A recent research study suggested that adding nicotinic acid to statin therapy was not associated with a lower risk of heart disease. These drugs work inside the intestine, where they bind to bile from the liver and prevent it from being reabsorbed into the circulatory system. Bile is made largely from cholesterol, so these drugs work by depleting the body's supply of cholesterol. The most common side effects are constipation, gas, and upset stomach.

Ezetimibe (Zetia) lowers bad LDL cholesterol by blocking cholesterol absorption in the intestine. Research studies have not found that ezetimibe is associated with a lower risk of heart disease.

Among the drugs that conflict with statins are hepatitis C protease inhibitors like telaprevir and boceprevir and the antibiotics erythromycin and clarithromycin.

Conclusion

Diabetes is on the rise and people are taking medications, yet people are not cured. In most cases, type 2 diabetes is preventable with healthy lifestyle changes. Sometimes it can even be reversed.

Taking steps to prevent and control diabetes doesn't mean living in deprivation. While eating right is important, you don't have to give up sweets entirely or resign yourself to a lifetime of bland health food. You can still enjoy your favorite foods and take pleasure from your meals without feeling hungry or deprived. However, you need to understand how to control the disease.

Have you recently been diagnosed with diabetes or prediabetes? Or has your doctor warned you that you're at risk? It can be scary to hear that your health's on the line, especially if you feel helpless to do anything about it.

Here's a scenario that may sound familiar: your doctor's telling you how important it is to lose weight and transform your eating habits, but you're already discouraged. After all, you've tried dieting in the past without success. And counting calories, measuring portion sizes, and following complicated food charts sounds like way too much work.

Whether you're trying to prevent or control diabetes, there is some good news. You can make a big difference with healthy lifestyle changes. The most important thing you can do for your health is to lose weight—and you don't have to lose all your extra pounds to reap the benefits. Experts say that losing just 5% to 10% of your total weight can help you lower your blood sugar considerably, as well as lower your blood pressure and cholesterol levels. It's not too late to make a positive change, even if you've already developed diabetes. The bottom line is that you have more control over your health than you think.

Eating right is vital if you're trying to prevent or control diabetes. While exercise is also important, what you eat has the biggest impact when it comes to weight loss. But what does eating right for diabetes mean? You may be surprised to hear that your nutritional needs are virtually the same as everyone else's: no special foods or complicated diets are necessary.

A diabetes diet is simply a healthy eating plan that is high in nutrients, low in fat, and moderate in calories. It is a healthy diet for anyone! The only difference is that you need to pay more attention to some of your food choices—most notably the carbohydrates you eat.

CHAPTER IX

Diabetes and Heart Disease

In this chapter we shall examine what constitutes diabetes and how it affects the heart, kidneys, and other parts of the body.

What Is Diabetes?

Diabetes is a condition in which the body does not properly process food for use as energy. Most of the food we eat is turned into glucose, or sugar, for our bodies to use for energy. The pancreas, an organ that lies near the stomach, makes a hormone called insulin to help glucose get into the cells of our bodies. When you have diabetes, your body either doesn't make enough insulin or can't use its own insulin as well as it should. This causes sugars to build up in your blood.

This is why many people refer to diabetes as "sugar." Diabetes can cause serious health complications including heart disease, blindness, kidney failure, and lower-extremity amputations. Diabetes is the seventh leading cause of death in the United States (Allo, Lincoln, Wilson, Green, Watanabe, Schaffer, 1991).

Diabetes among Black and Hispanic People

Black and Hispanic people love to fry their foods, and we eat a lot of carbohydrates, while many Asians and white people eat more vegetables and fruits. However, there are also many whites and Asians who eat junk foods. Therefore, among these people diabetes and heart disease rates are high. It is estimated that:

- Blacks are 1.7 times as likely to develop diabetes as whites.
- The prevalence of diabetes among blacks has quadrupled during the past 30 years.
- Among blacks age 20 and older in America, about 2.3 million have diabetes—0.8% of that age group.
- Blacks are more likely than non-Hispanic whites to develop diabetes and to experience greater disability from diabetes-related complications such as amputations, adult blindness, kidney failure, and increased risk of heart disease and stroke; Death rates for blacks with diabetes are 27% higher than for whites (Avogaro, Vigili de Kreutzenberg, Negut, Tiengo, Scognamiglio, 2004).

The way we eat and what we love to eat determine what kind of diseases we may suffer from if we do not change. This is part of the lifestyle we choose. Type 2 diabetes is often triggered by foods we eat and stress we experience. For those who have it, it can be controlled by diet and exercise. Your physician can you give you better guidelines, depending on your willingness to change your lifestyle. Left untreated, it will harm your body.

What Are the Symptoms of Diabetes?

People who think they might have diabetes must visit a physician for diagnosis. The following symptoms may be indications that you have diabetes:

- Frequent urination
- Excessive thirst
- Unexplained weight loss
- Extreme hunger
- Sudden vision changes
- Tingling or numbness in hands or feet
- Feeling very tired much of the time
- Very dry skin
- Sores that are slow to heal
- More infections than usual

- Nausea, vomiting, or stomach pains may accompany some of these symptoms in the abrupt onset of insulin-dependent diabetes, now called Type 1 diabetes

What Are the Types of Diabetes?

Type 1

Type 1 diabetes, previously called insulin-dependent diabetes mellitus (IDDM) or juvenile-onset diabetes, may account for 5-10% of all diagnosed cases of diabetes. Risk factors are less well defined for Type 1 diabetes than for Type 2 diabetes, but autoimmune, genetic, and environmental factors are involved in the development of this type of diabetes (Ruddy, Shumak, 1988). This disease starts early in life. Modification of diet helps. However, one has to take insulin to live because the pancreas is not able to produce any insulin.

Type 2

Type 2 diabetes was previously called non-insulin-dependent diabetes mellitus (NIDDM) or adult-onset diabetes. Type 2 diabetes may account for 90-95% of all diagnosed cases of diabetes. Risk factors for Type 2 diabetes include older age, obesity, family history of diabetes, prior history of gestational diabetes, impaired tolerance, physical inactivity, and race/ ethnicity. African Americans, Hispanic/Latino Americans, American Indians, and some Asian Americans and Pacific Islanders are at particularly high risk for type 2 diabetes (Ruddy, Shumak, 1988).

In this type of diabetes the body produces insulin, but not enough to open most receptor cells to bring in the nutrition they need. The glucose does not go into the cells, but goes around and around; blood sugar is high and yet the cells are starving in the midst of plenty of food. These receptors can be opened through exercise. If it is not enough, diabetic treatment can help to relieve the symptoms. The best solution is change of diet and exercise. Left untreated, type 2 diabetes can damage the kidneys and heart.

Gestational Diabetes

Gestational diabetes occurs more frequently in African Americans, Hispanic/Latino Americans, American Indians, and people with a family history of diabetes than in other groups. Obesity is also associated with higher risk. Women who have had gestational diabetes are at increased risk for later developing Type 2 diabetes.

In some studies, nearly 40% of women with a history of gestational diabetes developed diabetes in the future (Karvounis, Papadopoulos, Zaglavara, 2004).

Diabetic Cardiomyopathy

Diabetic cardiomyopathy (DCM) is a disorder of the heart muscle in people with diabetes. It can lead to inability of the heart to circulate blood through the body effectively, a state known as heart failure, with accumulation of fluid in the lungs (pulmonary edema) or legs (peripheral edema).

Most heart failure in people with diabetes results from coronary artery disease, and diabetic cardiomyopathy is only said to exist if there is no coronary artery disease to explain the heart muscle disorder (Avogaro, Vigili de Kreutzenberg, Negut, Tiengo, Scognamiglio, 2004).

One particularity of DCM is the long latent phase, during which the disease progresses but is completely asymptomatic. In most cases, DCM is detected with concomitant hypertension or coronary artery disease. One of the earliest signs is mild left ventricular diastolic dysfunction with little effect on ventricular filling.

Also, the diabetic patient may show subtle signs of DCM related to decreased left ventricular compliance or left ventricular hypertrophy or a combination of both. A prominent "a" wave can also be noted in the jugular venous pulse, and the cardiac apical impulse may be overactive or sustained throughout systole.

After the development of systolic dysfunction, left ventricular dilation, and symptomatic heart failure, the jugular venous pressure may become elevated, and the apical impulse would be displaced downward and to the left. Systolic mitral murmur is not uncommon in these cases. These changes are accompanied by a variety of electrocardiographic changes that may be associated with DCM in 60% of patients without structural heart disease, although usually not in the early asymptomatic phase (Aasum, Hafstad, Severson, Larsen, 2003).

Later in the progression, a prolonged QT interval may be indicative of fibrosis. Given that DCM's definition excludes concomitant atherosclerosis or hypertension, there are no changes in perfusion or in atrial natriuretic peptide levels up until the very late stages of the disease, when the hypertrophy and fibrosis become very pronounced.

Diabetic cardiomyopathy is characterized functionally by ventricular dilation, myocyte hypertrophy, prominent interstitial fibrosis, and decreased or preserved systolic function in the presence of a diastolic dysfunction.

While it has been evident for a long time that the complications seen in diabetes are related to the hyperglycemia associated with it, several factors have been implicated in the pathogenesis of the disease.

Etiologically, four main causes are responsible for the development of heart failure in DCM: microangiopathy and related endothelial dysfunction, autonomic neuropathy, metabolic alterations that include abnormal glucose use and increased fatty acid oxidation, generation and accumulation of free radicals, and alterations in ion homeostasis, especially calcium transients (Aasum, Hafstad, Severson, Larsen, 2003).

There is no single clinically effective treatment for diabetic cardiomyopathy. Treatment centers around intense glycemic control through diet, oral hypoglycemics and frequently insulin, and management of heart failure symptoms.

There is a clear correlation between increased glycemia and risk of developing diabetic cardiomyopathy; therefore, keeping glucose concentrations as controlled as possible is paramount. Thiazolidinediones are not recommended in patients with NYHA Class III or IV heart failure secondary to fluid retention (Davis, Fortun, Mulder, Davis, Bruce, 2004).

As with most other heart diseases, angiotensin-converting enzyme (ACE) inhibitors can also be administered. An analysis of major clinical trials shows that diabetic patients with heart failure benefit from such a therapy to a similar degree as non-diabetics. Similarly, beta blockers are also common in the treatment of heart failure concurrently with ACE inhibitors (Davis, Fortun, Mulder, Davis, Bruce, 2004).

Microangiopathy

Microangiopathy can be characterized as subendothelial and endothelial fibrosis in the coronary microvasculature of the heart. This endothelial dysfunction leads to impaired myocardial blood flow reserve as evidenced by echocardiography.

About 50% of diabetics with DCM show pathologic evidence for microangiopathy such as sub-endothelial and endothelial fibrosis, compared to only 21% of non-diabetic heart failure patients (Buse, Ginsberg, Bakris, 2007).

Over the years, several hypotheses were postulated to explain the endothelial dysfunction observed in diabetes. It was hypothesized that the extracellular hyperglycemia leads to an intracellular hyperglycemia in cells unable to regulate their glucose uptake, most predominantly endothelial cells. Indeed, while hepatocytes and myocytes have mechanisms allowing them to internalize their glucose transporter, endothelial cells do not possess this ability.

The consequences of increased intracellular glucose concentration are fourfold, all resulting from increasing concentration of glycolytic intermediates upstream of the rate-limiting glyceraldehyde-3-phosphate reaction which is inhibited by mechanisms activated by increased free radical formation, common in diabetes. Four pathways, enumerated below, explain part of the diabetic complications (Cesario Shivkumar, 2006).

- First, it has been widely reported since the 1960s that hyperglycemia causes an increase in the flux through aldose reductase and the polyol pathway. Increased activity of the detoxifying aldose reductase enzyme leads to a depletion of the essential cofactor NADH, thereby disrupting crucial cell processes.
- Second, increasing fructose 6-phosphate, a glycolysis intermediate, will lead to increased flux through the hexosamine pathway. This produces N-acetyl glucosamine that can add on serine and threonine residues and alter signaling pathways as well as cause pathological induction of certain transcription factors.
- Third, hyperglycemia causes an increase in diacylglycerol, which is also an activator of the protein kinase C (PKC) signaling pathway.

Induction of PKC causes multiple deleterious effects, including but not limited to blood flow abnormalities, capillary occlusion, and pro-inflammatory gene expression.

- Finally, glucose, as well as other intermediates such as fructose and glyceraldehyde-3-phosphate, when present in high concentrations, promote the formation of advanced glycation endproducts (AGEs). These, in turn, can irreversibly cross-link to proteins and cause intracellular aggregates that cannot be degraded by proteases and thereby, alter intracellular signaling. Also, AGEs can be exported to the intercellular space where they can bind AGE receptors (RAGE).

- This AGE/RAGE interaction activates inflammatory pathways such as NF-κB, in the host cells in an autocrine fashion, or in macrophages in a paracrine fashion. Neutrophil activation can also lead to NAD(P)H oxidase production of free radicals, further damaging the surrounding cells. Finally, exported glycation products bind extracellular proteins, alter the matrix and cell-matrix interactions, and promote fibrosis. A major source of increased myocardial stiffness is cross-linking between AGEs and collagen. In fact, a hallmark of uncontrolled diabetes is glycated products in the serum, which can be used as a marker for diabetic microangiopathy (Cesario, 2006).

Myocardial Metabolic Abnormalities

Possibly one of the first differences noticed in diabetic hearts was metabolic derangement. Indeed, even in the 1950s, it was recognized that cardiac myocyte from a diabetic patient had an abnormal, energy-inefficient metabolic function, with almost no carbohydrate oxidation (Chatham, Forder, 1997).

The changes seen in DCM are not dissimilar to those of ischemia, and might explain why diabetics are more susceptible to ischemic damage and are not easily preconditioned. Further, diabetes leads to persistent hyperglycemia very often accompanied by hyperlipidemia. This alters substrate availability to the heart and surely affects its metabolism.

Under normal conditions, fatty acids are the preferred substrate in the adult myocardium, supplying up to 70% of total ATP. They are oxidized in the mitochondrial matrix by the process of fatty acid β-oxidation, whereas pyruvate derived from glucose, glycogen, lactate and exogenous pyruvate is oxidized by the pyruvate dehydrogenase complex, localized within the inner mitochondrial membrane. Substrate choice in the adult heart is mainly regulated by availability, energy demand, and oxygen supply (the Randle cycle/glucose fatty-acid cycle).

Therefore, it is not surprising that alterations are present in diabetes and contribute greatly to its pathogenesis. Cardiomyocytes, unlike endothelial cells, have the ability to regulate their glucose uptake (Charonis, Reger, Dege, 1990). Thus, they are mostly spared from the complications associated with hyperglycemia that plague endothelial cells. In order to protect themselves from extracellular hyperglycemia, cardiac cells can internalize their insulin-dependent glucose transporter, GLUT4. When looking at the carbohydrate utilization of the myocardium, diabetic hearts not only show a decrease in glucose utilization but also a very pronounced decrease in lactate utilization, to a greater extent than glucose utilization (Choi, Zhong, Hoit, 2002). The mechanisms are unclear but are not related to lactate transport or lactate dehydrogenase expression. Further, due to a deficient carbohydrate uptake, the diabetic myocardium shows increases in intracellular glycogen pool, possibly through augmented synthesis or decreased glycogenolysis.

However, as a downside to this decrease glucose uptake, cardiomyocytes are faced with a reduced glucose oxidation rate and a dramatically increased fatty acid β-oxidation to almost 100% of ATP production. This is translated into a dramatic increase of fatty acid transporter, especially CD36, which is postulated to have an important role in the etiology of cardiac disease. Interestingly, it seems that the decrease in carbohydrate oxidation precedes the appearance of hyperglycemia in type 2 diabetes (Clerk, Rattigan, Clark, 2002).

It is likely due to the increased β-oxidation due to the hyperlipidemia and altered insulin signaling. The rate of uptake of lipids, unlike that of glucose, is not regulated by a hormone. Therefore, increased circulating lipids will increase uptake and thereby fatty acid oxidation. This, in turn, increases the concentration of citrate in the cell, a very potent inhibitor of phosphofructokinase, the first rate-limiting step of glycolysis. When the rate of uptake is greater than the rate of oxidation, fatty acids are shuttled to the triglyceride synthesis pathway. Increasing triglyceride stores prevents lipotoxicity but decreases heart function.

Why are all those alterations detrimental to the heart? Emerging evidence supports the concept that alterations in metabolism contribute to cardiac contractile dysfunction. In animal models, contractile failure begins as a diastolic dysfunction, and progresses occasionally to systolic dysfunction ultimately leading to heart failure.

Normalizing energy metabolism in these hearts reversed the impaired contractility. During diabetes, metabolic remodeling precedes the cardiomyopathy and it is valid to hypothesize that these changes may contribute to cardiac dysfunction. Indeed, when treating animal models with metabolic modulators at an early age, prior to any sign of cardiomyopathy, improvements of heart function can be noted .

While the heart can function without help from the nervous system, it is highly innervated with autonomic nerves, regulating the heartbeat according to demand in a fast manner, prior to hormonal release. The autonomic innervations of the myocardium in DCM are altered and contribute to myocardial dysfunction.

Unlike the brain, the peripheral nervous system does not benefit from a barrier protecting it from the circulating levels of glucose. Just like endothelial cells, nerve cells cannot regulate their glucose uptake and suffer the same types of damage listed above.

Therefore, the diabetic heart shows clear denervation as the pathology progresses. This denervation correlates with echocardiographic evidence of diastolic dysfunction and results in a decline of survival in patients with diabetes from 85% to 44%. Other causes of denervation are ischemia from microvascular disease, which appears following the development of microangiopathy (Mallinson, 2010).

Unlike most other cell types, the heart has constantly and rapidly changing ionic status, with various ion currents going in out of the cell during each beat cycle. More importantly, calcium is a major player in cardiac electromechanical events, energy metabolism, and contractile function. It moves across the sarcolemma, sarcoplasmic reticulum, and mitochondrial membranes through various organelle-specific channels by active transport as well as passive diffusion. Around 30-40% of the ATP production of a cardiomyocyte is primarily used by the sarcoplasmic reticulum Ca2+-ATPase (SERCA) and other ion pumps.

Thus, it is evident that any alteration in homeostasis will have serious consequences for the heart's function and possibly its integrity and structure. In DCM, such alterations have been noted since the late 1980s. Indeed, studies indicate a decrease in the ability of the cell to remove Ca2+ through Na+-Ca2+exchange and Ca2+-pump systems in the sarcolemma of diabetic rat hearts. More recently, decreased SERCA activity was shown to be a major contributor to the development of cardiac dysfunction in diabetes and decreased expression of the channel was also reported (Choi, Zhong, Hoit, 2002).

These differences are partly explained by altered calcium signaling at the level of the ryanodine receptor, a key regulator of SERCA, as well as increases in phospholamban observed in diabetic hearts. Originally, these abnormalities were thought to be associated with intracellular calcium overload; however, subsequent evidence blames altered [Ca2+]i transients with unchanged basal concentrations.

These alterations are not limited to calcium currents. Increases in intracellular sodium concentrations also play a causative role in ischemic damage sensitivity in diabetes and are related to a decrease in the Na+-H+ pump activity due to hyperglycemia. Furthermore, there is a decrease in Na+-K+ ATPase subunit expression, correlating with a decrease in expression of the Na+-Ca2+ exchanger.

More importantly, several potassium current abnormalities are observed. DCM causes alterations in transcription and surface expression of potassium channel proteins, which are theorized to be under the control of the insulin-signaling cascade. Indeed, abnormalities in K+ can be restored *in vitro* following incubation with insulin. Further, altered duration of the action potential, known to be increased in DCM, was shown to result mainly from a decreased K+ transmembrane permeability (Choi, Zhong, Hoit, 2002).

The Best Solutions for Diabetic People

As maintained before in this chapter, natural remedies and natural foods may be the best solutions for diabetic people. The Chinese and Egyptians used cinnamon as a remedy for high blood sugar for centuries. Cinnamon also is known to reduce high cholesterol, relieve arthritis pain, and fight cancer. Whenever my blood sugar is high from stress or eating foods high in carbohydrates, I have used cinnamon to reduce it. In fact, it has been the best treatment I have ever experienced. I do not feel any side effects as I used to do when taking medications for nearly 10 years.

Cinnamon

It is believed that cinnamon was one of the commercial products sold in Egypt as early as 2,000 BC. Cinnamon was sold from Ethiopia, Sri Lanka, Arabia, China, and north India.

It is theorized that this herbal remedy can reduce insulin resistance in people with type 2 diabetes and help the body to control sugar level. There was a study done in China which concluded that if cinnamon was taken in ground form, it reduced blood sugar level in people with type 2 diabetes. (This research was done at the Clinical Medical College of Jiangsu University on 66 patients.) I can attest that I am number 67. This herbal remedy works better than any other type 2 diabetes medication on the market. I believe in it and I can recommend it to anyone with type 2 diabetes.

The experiment was done for three months with the 66 diabetic patients. The end result was that after three months, patients' fasting blood glucose levels were lower and hemoglobin improved. The same study was done at the University of California and showed better results with patients with pre-diabetes. However, "although these and other studies have found similar results, the American Diabetes Association does not acknowledge cinnamon as a diabetes treatment based on limitations of the research" (Reeder, 2014).

Even though the American Diabetes Association has not acknowledged cinnamon as a treatment for diabetes, based on my personal experience with the remedy, I conclude that it has worked for me. It is up to you to try it or not. I am only sharing what works for me.

Is Cinnamon Safe?

Cinnamon supplements are classified as a food, not a drug, and are not subject to the same safety and effectiveness tests as medications. Also, because cinnamon can lower blood sugar levels, you should be cautious about combining it with medications intended to do the same. It is always better to talk to your doctor before trying an herbal remedy to treat your diabetes. This will help you to have peace of mind (Reeder, 2014).

Conclusion

After going through this chapter, you have seen how diabetes affects people's health. It does not discriminate; it does not choose whom to affect and not to affect. Any one of us can have this disease.

I suggest that the solution to conquer this disease is not in medicine, but in changing lifestyle, changing diet, and being active daily. However, as we have seen, with type 1 diabetes and gestational diabetes, you may need insulin when necessary.

You need to work with your physician on your treatment. I do not suggest that you take these matters into your own hands.

Before I was diagnosed with type 2 diabetes, I had all the symptoms mentioned in this chapter. I had no energy to do anything. All I wanted was to drink a lot of water and sleep. My wife thought I was too lazy; she did not understand and I did not understand myself what was going on in my body. God protected me from car accidents many times because I would be driving half awake and half asleep. Now I know how diabetes can affect your body.

CHAPTER X
How to Remain Healthy

Everyone wants to be healthy, but healthy lives do not come freely. It takes discipline and maintenance. You may ask, "How do I get a healthier heart right now?" The answer sounds too good to be true: By simply living a healthier lifestyle. Heart disease is preventable and studies have shown that 90% of heart attacks in women can be prevented.

Furthermore, the latest study indicates that changes in your lifestyle mean a stronger, more efficient heart. The Archives of Internal Medicine shows that women who eat veggies, fruit, whole grains, fish, and legumes; do not drink alcohol; exercise; maintain a healthy weight; and don't smoke have a 92% lower risk of a heart attack compared with women with less healthy diets and habits.

I would exclude fish because even if fish has omega-3, you can get omega-3 in plant foods, such as sesame seeds. Alcohol is never good for anyone. However, people make medical excuses so they can continue to consume what they like and enjoy. They end up paying in their later years, if not very soon.

There are so many things we can do to help our hearts remain healthy, like quitting smoking and eating more fiber. Moving more also help other parts of our body, including your bones, colon, lungs and skin. Doctors usually talk about good and bad cholesterol and most folks will have that down, but triglycerides are a better marker for high risk of diabetes and heart disease.

Triglycerides are also much more responsive to lifestyle changes than other types of blood fats. You can lower triglycerides 30% to 50% just by reducing saturated fats and reducing your weight. Your heart will love you if you eat six walnuts before lunch and dinner. Why? Because "walnuts are rich in omega-3 fatty acids, which help to decrease inflammation in the arteries surrounding your heart, so they keep your heart functioning longer and better. Walnuts will also make you feel fuller faster so you are less likely to overeat at meals." This will be better than consuming eggs that cause accumulation of cholesterol in your body. Probably, this is a solution for people who eat more than 2,000 calories a day.

What we eat affects the formation of neurotransmitters, and some diet-related neurotransmitters have a significant effect on mood, appetite, and cravings. This in turn causes the brain to communicate in the form of an impulse (craving for certain foods) the need for certain neurotransmitters that it requires to restore balance. While many other factors influence the levels of these chemicals, such as hormones, heredity, drugs, and alcohol, three neurotransmitters—dopamine, norepinephrine, and serotonin—have been studied in relation to food, and this research has shown that neurotransmitters are produced in the brain from components of certain foods. When your body has enough dopamine you're blessed with feelings of bliss and pleasure, focus, euphoria, appetite control, and controlled motor movements. When we are low in dopamine we feel no pleasure, our world looks colorless, we have an inability to "love," and we have no remorse about personal behavior.

The brain cells that "manufacture" dopamine use l-phenylalanine as a "raw material" (precursor). Phenylalanine is an essential amino acid found in the brain and blood plasma that can convert in the body to tyrosine, which in turn is used to synthesize dopamine. Sources of phenylalanine are high-protein foods such as beans and wheat germ. These are natural foods. Lovers of meat will say meat is the best source of phenylalanine, but meat is not the only high-protein food. Soybeans and other plant foods, such as legumes and peas, also have high protein the body needs.

Apples

A compound called quercetin, found in apples, is an antioxidant that studies have shown may not only help in the prevention of cancer but may also play an important role in the prevention of neurodegenerative disorders. People with Alzheimer's and dementia can benefit from this fruit. There may be something to that old saying, "An apple a day keeps the doctor away."

Bananas

Bananas are a good source of tyrosine. Tyrosine is the amino acid neurons turn into norepinephrine and dopamine. Norepinephrine and dopamine are excitatory neurotransmitters that are important in motivation, alertness, concentration, and memory. Bananas are also a good source of natural potassium that helps the heart to depolarize.

Beans and Legumes

Beans and legumes are rich in protein and are healthful boosters of both dopamine and norepinephrine. The benefit you get is the same found in meat, milk, eggs, cheese, fish, and other seafood.

Beets

Betaine, an amino acid naturally present in certain vegetables, particularly beets, is an antidepressant of the first order. Betaine acts as a stimulant for the production of SAM-e (S-adenoslmethionine). The body cannot do without SAM-e, which it produces. SAM-e is directly related to the production of certain hormones, such as dopamine and serotonin. As already stated, dopamine is responsible for feelings of well-being and pleasure.

Cheese

Cheese is high in protein and calcium. Protein provides amino acids, which help produce dopamine and norepinephrine. However, you should not consume too much cheese. You can get norepinephrine from other natural sources with less effect on your health.

Chicken

Chicken, like eggs, contains complete protein that increases levels of the excitatory neurotransmitters norepinephrine and dopamine. Chicken is also a good source of coenzyme Q10, which increases the energy-generating potential of neurons. However, I would not recommend eating too much chicken meat. If you have to eat chicken, roasted or baked is better than fried. Male chickens are better than female chickens, because females hold a lot of fats for producing eggs.

Cottage Cheese

One of the "must eat" foods on every expert's list, cottage cheese is recommended as a substitute for other soft cheeses and dairy products. Cottage cheese provides the protein that can help boost mood and energy levels, without some of the fat of hard cheeses.

Again, not too much cheese is needed for your body; you can live with it, but there are other sources of what you can get from cheese.

Research from the University of California, Berkeley suggests that people who suffer from depression have low amounts of serotonin, norepinephrine, and dopamine in their brains. One natural antidepressant is to increase dopamine by eating protein-rich foods such as eggs or cheese, because they are versatile and appeal to some people who choose not to eat meat.

Fish

Omega-3 fatty acids are found in seafood, especially mackerel, salmon, striped bass, rainbow trout, halibut, tuna, and sardines. For vegetarians, there are plant foods that can provide the same benefits. These fatty acids may have many jobs in the body, including a possible role in the production of neurotransmitters. Fish have easily digestible protein, many trace nutrients, high quality essential fatty acids, low cholesterol levels, and low saturated fat levels. Some have shown that rats deficient in omega-3 fatty acids had more receptors for the neurotransmitter serotonin and a corresponding decrease in dopamine in the frontal cortex. Find a substitute for fish if you are like me and do not eat fish.

Watermelon

Watermelon juice is fat-free and loaded with vitamins A, B6, and C! The body uses Vitamin B6 to manufacture neurotransmitters such as serotonin, melatonin, and dopamine. Vitamin C enhances the immune system while protecting the body from free radicals. It also tastes good, right?

Wheat Germ

Wheat germ is a good source of phenylalanine. Phenylalanine is an essential amino acid found in the brain and blood plasma that can convert in the body to tyrosine, which in turn is used to synthesize dopamine.

A healthy, balanced diet is rich in whole "natural" and unprocessed foods. It is especially high in plant foods, such as fruits, vegetables, grains, beans, seeds, and nuts. Fruits and vegetables are rich in fiber, vitamins, minerals, and antioxidants that protect the body cells from damage. They also help raise serotonin levels in the brain.

These foods above are beneficial to your health; however, I would be careful with animal foods. Eggs are known to increase cholesterol. Some cholesterol is good for your body but one egg per week may be enough for your health. Chicken is also an animal product, and consuming too much of it can cause problems. If you cannot live without it, eat skinless chicken, baked or roasted. These methods help to reduce fats in the chicken.

Fish has omega-3. Keep in mind that some nuts and seeds can give you similar results. If you cannot live without animal flesh, fish or chicken would be better than red meat. However, I would recommend that you eat natural plant foods. You may end up paying back with your life, If you eat too much chicken meat. Natural plant foods are good for your heart and the rest of your body. There is no hard cholesterol in most plant foods. Some, like palm oils, do have cholesterol, although it is not as bad as animal fats.

It is widely believed that vegetable oils such as olive oil clean your blood vessels while animal fats plug the vessels and arteries. Thus, it is best to eat plant oils instead of oils from animal fats.

Benefits of Running and Walking

It is widely believed that walking or running have similar results in lowering the risk of heart disease. A brisk walk may be just as good as a run for keeping the heart healthy. That's encouraging, considering less than half of Americans meet the government's recommendation of at least 2.5 hours of moderate to intense aerobic exercise a week (Shimoni, Ewart, Severson, 1999).

A study published in the American Heart Association (AHA) journal *Arteriosclerosis, Thrombosis and Vascular Biology* found that walkers lowered their risk of high blood pressure, high cholesterol, and diabetes as much as runners. Researchers studied 33,060 runners who were participating in the National Runners' Health Study and 15,045 walkers enrolled in the National Walkers' Health Study over six years. All the participants were between the ages of 18 and 80, with most in their 40s and 50s. The exercises answered questionnaires about their physical activity, and the researchers calculated how much energy they expended based on the distance the volunteers reported walking or running. They also recorded any doctor-diagnosed heart conditions (Magyar, Cseresnyés, Rusznák, Sipos, Szücs, Kovács, 1995).

The scientists found that while vigorous running required slightly higher levels of energy than moderate-intensity walking, both translated into a parallel drop in incidence of high blood pressure, high cholesterol, diabetes, or heart disease over the study period. And the more the participants walked or ran, the greater the benefit in lowering their heart disease risk.

Although walking isn't as intense as running, the study authors say both target the same muscle groups, which could explain why their results in improving heart health are so similar. The results suggest that the type of exercise may not be as important as how much people walk or run.

Here's what the researchers found:

- Running significantly reduced the risk for being diagnosed with hypertension by 4.2%, while walking reduced the risk by 7.2%
- Running reduced the chances of having high cholesterol by 4.3% and walking by 7%
- Running lowered risk of diabetes by 12.1%, while walking dropped the risk by 12.3%
- Running reduced coronary heart disease risk by 4.5%, compared to 9.3% for walking

The results are encouraging, since walking may be more appealing and sustainable for more people than running. Because running is a more intense form of physical activity, runners are able to burn more calories and exercise the heart to higher levels within a shorter period of time, but the results support the idea that any physical activity, as long as it's consistent, can have lasting benefits (Jourdon, Feuvray, 1993)

Conclusion

Improving your heart health by improving your diet may not be drastically difficult, though your new diet will be lacking in extremely salty, sugary, or fatty foods.

Health workers advise limiting portions of the foods you eat to a reasonable size and eating several small meals during the day instead of two or three large meals per day. A variety of fruits and vegetables are important, along with lean meat and dairy. Legumes (beans) and fish are essential because they contain disease-fighting ingredients including vitamins, minerals, and omega-3 fatty acids. Eating raw vegetables and minimally cooked food is a good addition to your diet because it helps preserve necessary enzymes.

Salt intake should be very low as well. Flaxseed oil is extremely good for your health and heart because it has essential fatty acids. Garlic and onion are necessary in your diet because they provide antioxidants and lower cholesterol and triglycerides.

When choosing foods for heart health, don't just consider fat and calories, but sugar content too, especially if you have elevated blood sugar. Potatoes can be a healthy part of a meal even for people who've had a heart attack. However, if potatoes make your blood sugar skyrocket, you should avoid eating them. High blood sugar leads to lots of insulin in your veins, which can damage your arteries and contribute to a heart attack.

The foods you eat can directly and substantially affect your heart. If you have high cholesterol, a diet should be aimed at lowering it. Heart attack and cholesterol levels are linked. High blood pressure calls for a hypertension diet that probably cuts back on fat and restricts salt. Some people thrive on the protein-rich, low-carbohydrate diet.

Diet therapy for heart patients is a big part of recovery after a heart attack. For heart attack patients and people with heart problems, a recipe for heart health includes preventing another heart attack, eating wholesome ingredients, and at least moderate exercise.

Taking more pills does not mean we have less heart disease, less high blood pressure, or lower cholesterol. In fact, the opposite seems to be true. If you are medicated or thinking that is your only option, that will only be the beginning of possible health care crises you will have. Medical expenses are extremely high, and while quality goes down they will continue to increase.

Another factor to consider is the lack of exercise in our lives. In the western world, there is too much sitting in our cars, and too much watching television. There is also a problem with the foods we eat. We either eat too much or eat animal foods that are hard for the body to process in large amounts.

God allowed animal foods during the flood. However, we have made this our permanent diet. If people were to eat raw vegetables and fruits and nuts, health care would be under control. The number one killer (heart disease) would lose the market. As long as we continue to consume animal foods, we will continue to depend on heart and cholesterol medication. Sickness will continue and life will be either short or full of pain and disease. That is a result of not following God's health principles.

It is my hope that this book will bring you health awareness and help you to make a better choice for your health and life. Remember, not everything that tastes good is good for your health. The factors above can be avoided and you will not have to suffer with heart disease. Again, this is a choice you have to make for yourself and your family. The solution to the heart problem is in your hands. Obesity is mostly caused by eating more than what the body needs. You can control it by reducing the calories you eat, reducing stress, eating more fiber, and exercising daily.

Depending on medication to treat heart disease does not solve the problem. Medications treat symptoms; it is up to you to change the way you eat and live. Even in old age, heart disease can be controlled, I therefore encourage you to change your lifestyle and live a healthy life free from heart disease.

As you can see in this chapter, it is not necessary to eat animal foods. There are vegetarian foods you can eat and get even better benefits.

Our choice of fats and oils is extremely important; most people, especially infants and growing children, benefit from more fat in the diet. But the fats we eat must be chosen with care. Avoid all processed foods containing newfangled hydrogenated fats and polyunsaturated oils. Instead, use traditional vegetable oils like extra virgin olive oil and small amounts of unrefined flax seed oil. Organic butter, extra virgin olive oil, and expeller-expressed flax oil in opaque containers are available in health food stores and gourmet markets. They are all good for your heart.

CHAPTER XI

Food and Your Heart

Someone said, "we are what we eat." Today, there are higher numbers of young patients afflicted by high blood pressure, high cholesterol, diabetes, and heart disease. Conventionally, these are disorders of age, likely to develop in the fifth or sixth decade of one's life. But poor eating habits and lack of physical exercise are bringing on an epidemic of these diseases. The patient profile is getting younger every day.

Over the past few decades, the diet pattern in the USA and the world has drastically changed. The dietary choices of individuals in India used to be based on tradition, culture, and religious beliefs, but now convenience is the rule of thumb. Convenience food is quick, tasty, and (very importantly) "fashionable." Lack of time to exercise, stress, and boredom are the most common excuses my patients give for indulging in such foods. I wonder what will be the end result for this generation.

Hamburger

This is not a good food for the heart; it is high in fat as well as bad cholesterol, which affects your heart. I always counsel people who like to eat meat to eat white meat instead of red meat. By white meat I mean chicken and turkey.

Every time we eat unhealthy foods, we are digging our own early graves slowly. By the time we have eaten enough, we are ready to get into the graves we dug by ourselves. At this point medical interventions are not the solution to keep us alive (White, 2007).

Eggs

Eggs do have high cholesterol, which is not good for the heart. If possible, do not consume more than necessary. If you're diagnosed with high cholesterol or you are diabetic, it is better to avoid them all together.

Exercising and eating raw foods will give you vitamin take away some of the toxicity, which may reduce accumulations of cholesterol in your blood streams. May be is the best way to better healthy lives.

Fried Foods

Chips smell good and taste good as well, but they are very dangerous to your heart. This is true of all fried foods. They are bad for your heart. They may taste good, but the end result is bad.

Restaurant Food and Junk Food

Dining out is an easier option for overworked professionals than cooking at home these days. While the frequency of eating out at restaurants has zoomed, so have portion sizes. People consume more calories now than ever before.

Skipping breakfast, heavy dinners, long gaps between meals; lack of fiber-rich food is so very evident in the diets of today's world economy. And it's a trend that starts early. Children are introduced to junk food at a very young age and very soon chips, cold drinks, biscuits, pizzas, burgers, box juices, and a whole host of unwholesome foods become a major part of their everyday diet.

Let's not just blame busy professionals, double-income families, or working mothers. The prevalence of television commercials promoting unhealthy food as healthy and nutritious has contributed a lot to poor eating habits. Consumption of cold drinks, especially among children, for instance, has increased in the last 20 years by 300%. Children have become more sedentary, and outdoor sports have taken a backseat. Lack of physical activity, increasing affluence, and easy availability of fast and convenient foods lead to obesity and ultimately risk of heart disease.

Foods from different parts of the world are now just a phone call away in any metro. We often label Western pizzas and burgers as "junk food," but Indian fast foods such as chat, samosa, namkeen, and traditional sweets are equally loaded with calories and saturated fat. If trans fatty acids in high-fat baked foods like doughnuts, cookies, cakes, rusks, and biscuits clog your arteries, so do saturated fats in cream, cheese, butter, and ghee hidden in Indian snacks.

Processed foods containing partially hydrogenated vegetable oils should be avoided. They are rich sources of fat. They increase bad cholesterol (or LDL), bring down good cholesterol (HDL), and are more prone to getting deposited in blood vessels, leading to heart attacks and stroke.

Cardiovascular disease is the single most important cause of deaths worldwide. High blood pressure, high cholesterol, diabetes, obesity, sedentary lifestyle, and a diet rich in saturated fats—especially processed and ready-to-eat foods—are the major risk factors that lead to various heart ailments. All of these can be controlled through a healthy diet and lifestyle.

Although you might know that eating certain foods can increase your heart disease risk, it's often tough to change your eating habits. How much you eat is just as important as what you eat. Overloading your plate, taking seconds, and eating until you feel stuffed can lead to eating more calories, fat, and cholesterol than you should. Portions served in restaurants are often more than anyone needs. Keep track of the number of servings you eat—and use proper serving sizes—to help control your portions. Eating more of low-calorie, nutrient-rich foods, such as fruits and vegetables, and less of high-calorie, high-sodium foods, such as refined, processed, or fast foods, can shape up your diet as well as your heart and waistline.

People who have extra weight on them eat more than their share or more than the body can use. It is stored in the form of fat in the tissues. I am not trying to attack people who have extra weight on them. I know this is a struggle for most people. It is easier to gain weight than lose it. This has to do with our lifestyle and what we eat.

A serving size is a specific amount of food, defined by common measurements such as cups, ounces or pieces. For example, one serving of pasta is 1/2 cup, or about the size of a hockey puck. A serving of meat, fish, or chicken is two to three ounces, or about the size and thickness of a deck of cards. Judging serving size is a learned skill. You may need to use measuring cups and spoons or a scale until you're comfortable with your judgment.

If you like eating, eating more vegetables is better than eating refined low-fiber food that takes a lot of time to leave the GI tract. The more food stays in the GI tract, the easier it is to gain weight. So what should we do about obesity? The solution is easy and simple. Eat food with a lot of fiber, such as fruits and vegetables. Stay away from animal fats. Exercise daily and watch what goes into your mouth. You will be happy with the end results.

Vegetables and Fruits

Vegetables and fruits are good sources of vitamins and minerals. They are also low in calories and rich in dietary fiber, and contain substances that may help prevent cardiovascular disease. Eating more fruits and vegetables may help you eat less high-fat foods, such as meat, cheese, and snack foods.

Fruits and vegetables to choose	Fruits and vegetables to avoid
Fresh or frozen vegetables and fruits	Coconut
Low-sodium canned vegetables	Vegetables with creamy sauces
Canned fruit packed in juice or water	Fried or breaded vegetables
	Canned fruit packed in heavy syrup
	Frozen fruit with sugar added

Featuring vegetables and fruits in your diet can be easy. Keep vegetables washed and cut in your refrigerator for quick snacks. Keep fruit in a bowl in your kitchen so that you'll remember to eat it. Choose recipes that have vegetables or fruits as the main ingredient, such as vegetable stir-fry or fresh fruit mixed into salads.

Select Whole Grains

Whole grains are good sources of fiber and other nutrients that play a role in regulating blood pressure and heart health.

Grain products to choose	Grain products to limit or avoid
Whole-wheat flour	White, refined flour
Whole-grain bread, preferably	White bread
100% whole-wheat bread or 100%	Muffins
whole-grain bread	Frozen waffles
High-fiber cereal with 5 g or more	Corn bread
of fiber in a serving	Doughnuts
Whole grains such as brown rice,	Biscuits
barley and buckwheat (kasha)	Quick breads
Whole-grain pasta	Granola bars
Oatmeal (steel-cut or regular)	Cakes
Ground flaxseed	Pies
	Egg noodles
	Buttered popcorn
	High-fat snack crackers

You can increase the amount of whole grains in a heart-healthy diet by making simple substitutions for refined grain products. Or be adventuresome and try a new whole grain, such as whole-grain couscous, quinoa, or barley.

Another easy way to add whole grains to your diet is ground flaxseed. Flaxseeds are small brown seeds that are high in fiber and omega-3 fatty acids, which can lower your total blood cholesterol. You can grind the seeds in a coffee grinder or food processor and stir a teaspoon of them into yogurt, applesauce, or hot cereal.

Fats

Limiting the saturated and trans fats you eat is an important step to reduce your blood cholesterol and lower your risk of coronary artery disease. High blood cholesterol can lead to a buildup of plaques in your arteries, called atherosclerosis, which can increase your risk of heart attack and stroke. The American Heart Association offers these guidelines for how much fat and cholesterol to include in a heart-healthy diet:

Type of fat	Recommendation
Saturated fat	Less than 7% of your total daily calories, or less than 14 g of saturated fat if you follow a 2,000-calorie-a-day diet
Trans fat	Less than 1% of your total daily calories, or less than 2 g of trans fat if you follow a 2,000-calorie-a-day diet
Cholesterol	Less than 300 mg a day for healthy adults; less than 200 mg a day for adults with high levels of LDL ("bad") cholesterol or those who are taking cholesterol-lowering medication

The best way to reduce saturated and trans fats in your diet is to limit the amount of solid fats—butter, margarine, and shortening—you add to food when cooking and serving. You can also reduce the amount of saturated fat in your diet by trimming fat off your meat or choosing lean meats with less than 10% fat. You can also use low-fat substitutions when possible for a heart-healthy diet. For example, top your baked potato with salsa or low-fat yogurt rather than butter, or use low-sugar fruit spread on your toast instead of margarine.

You may also want to check the food labels of some cookies, crackers, and chips. Many of these snacks—even those labeled "reduced fat"—may be made with oils containing trans fats. One clue that a food has some trans fat in it is the phrase "partially hydrogenated" in the ingredient list.

When you do use fats, choose monounsaturated fats, such as olive oil or canola oil. Polyunsaturated fats, found in nuts and seeds, also are good choices for a heart-healthy diet. When used in place of saturated fat, monounsaturated and polyunsaturated fats may help lower your total blood cholesterol. But moderation is essential. All types of fat are high in calories (Pereira, Matthes, Schuster, 2006).

Fats to choose	Fats to limit
Olive oil	Butter
Canola oil	Lard
Margarine that's free of trans fats	Bacon fat
Cholesterol-lowering margarine,	Gravy
such as Benecol, Promise Active or	Cream sauce
Smart Balance	Nondairy creamers
	Hydrogenated margarine and
	shortening.
	Cocoa butter, found in chocolate.
	Coconut, palm, cottonseed and
	palm-kernel oils.

Apples for Better Health

One medium-sized apple contains about four grams of fiber. Some of that is in the form of pectin, a type of soluble fiber that has been linked to lower levels of LDL or "bad" cholesterol. That's because it blocks absorption of cholesterol, according to WebMD, which helps the body to use it rather than store it. The wealth of fiber an apple provides keep you feeling full for longer without costing you a lot of calories—there are about 95 in a medium-sized piece of fruit. That's because it takes our bodies longer to digest complex fiber than more simple materials like sugar or refined grains. Anything with at least three grams of fiber is a good source of the nutrient; most people should aim to get about 25 to 40 grams a day.

One component of an apple's peel (which also has most of the fiber) is something called ursolic acid, which was linked to a lower risk of obesity in a recent study in mice. That's because it boosts calorie burn and increases muscle and brown fat. (Brown fats are essential for children to keep them warm.) You have also heard that "an apple a day keeps the doctor away," which actually is very true. Apples have enzymes which keep you happy and healthy.

Five or more apples a week (less than an apple a day!) has been linked with better lung function, most likely because of an antioxidant called quercetin found in the skin of apples (as well as in onions and tomatoes),

PHILIP J. RUSHEMEZA, MD., PHD.

the BBC reports. The breath benefits of apples extend even further: a 2007 study found that women who eat plenty of the fruit are less likely to have children with asthma (BBC, 2007).

While they don't quite rival oranges, apples are considered a good source of immune-system-boosting vitamin C, with over 8 milligrams per medium-sized fruit, which amounts to roughly 14% of your daily-recommended intake.

In 2004, French research found that a chemical in apples helped prevent colon cancer, WebMD reported. And in 2007, a study from Cornell University found additional compounds, called triterpenoids, which seem to fight against liver, colon, and breast cancers.

A 2012 study published in the *American Journal of Clinical Nutrition* found that apples, as well as pears and blueberries, were linked with a lower risk of developing type 2 diabetes because of a class of antioxidants, anthocyanins, that are also responsible for red, purple, and blue colors in fruits and veggies.

The fruit has been linked to an uptick in acetylcholine production, which communicates between nerve cells, so apples may help your memory and lower your chances of developing Alzheimer's (Pereira, Matthes, Schuster, 2006).

Conclusion

From breakfast to dinner (and snacks in between), your entire day can be heart-healthy! A good-for-your-ticker diet doesn't have to be bland or boring, as we show you here with these *heart*-y foods that will leave you satisfied. The multi-billion-dollar organic food industry is fueled by consumer perception that organic food is healthier (greater nutritional value and fewer toxic chemicals).

Start your day with a steaming bowl of oats, which are full of omega-3 fatty acids, folate, and potassium. This fiber-rich super food can lower levels of LDL (or bad) cholesterol and help keep arteries clear. Opt for coarse or steel-cut oats over instant varieties—which contain more fiber—and top your bowl off with a banana for another four grams of fiber.

"Natural" and "organic" are not interchangeable terms. You may see "natural" and other terms such as "all natural," "free-range," or "hormone-free" on food labels. These descriptions must be truthful, but don't confuse them with the term "organic." Only foods that are grown and processed according to USDA organic standards can be labeled organic (USDA, 2012).

These foods are good for us, better than drugs, which accumulate free radicals in our blood and organs. They clean free radicals from our bodies.

God said, "I have given you every plant yielding seeds that is upon the face of all the earth and every tree with seeds in its fruit; you shall have them for food" (Genesis 1:29 NRSV).

My family, pictured, enjoys eating fresh vegetables and fruits. You can eat as many as you want; it can only make you a healthy and happy person. They are full of vitamins A, C, and E, they are good for cleaning your blood, and they repair the liver and GI tract.

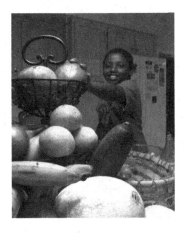

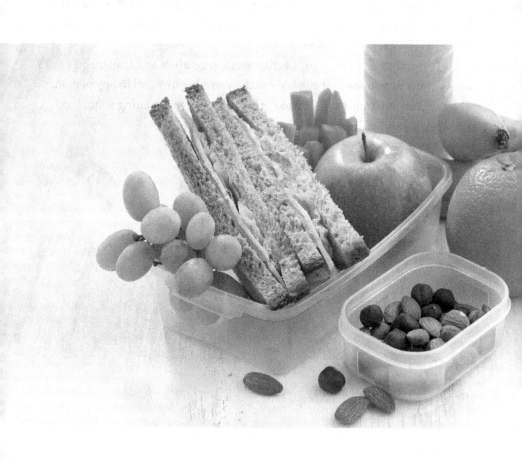

After reading this book, you might ask, "Why should anyone need a doctor? Does my physician have secret solutions to my health problems? Who has the last say on my physical body? Who controls my well-being?"

As a physician, I would say that physicians care about and want to help the patients they see every day. However, there comes a time when a physician can do nothing more to save someone's life. It is heartbreaking. Some patients seek help when it is no longer possible to reverse the physical damage. Others know they have a health problem but continue to follow an unhealthy lifestyle and expect their physicians to fix it all when symptoms get worse.

After a patient has passed away, physicians always wonder if there was something else we could have done to save that life. It is always joyous when physicians are able to use their medical training to save patients' lives, but in many cases there is nothing we can do to reverse the patient's situation. It is very difficult in medical practice when a physician tries everything to save a life, yet is blamed for not succeeding.

Most physicians went into the medical field to make a difference in people's lives, but as much as we might try to treat and save lives, better health largely relies on each individual's choice and not on a physician's ability to cure.

If patients come to the physician for heart disease, yet continue to smoke or eat unhealthy foods, can they expect miracles to reverse a damaged heart? In this case, a physician cannot be the solution to better health. The solution to a better healthy life without cardiovascular disease, type 2 diabetes, or cancer is available to each one of us. God gives us health laws so we may remain healthy and free from diseases (Leviticus 11). We can only remain healthy if we follow God's health principles.

Do you realize that in the Garden of Eden, God did not give Adam and Eve animal foods for consumption? God gave them plants. In fact, there were fruits of all kinds that provided all the nutrition. Adam and Eve ate fruit and their lives were without disease and death. When they disobeyed God and started eating animal foods, stress and disease came upon them. Their bodies started breaking down, and they died.

God told them on the day they disobeyed his command that they would surely die. Adam lived for about 930 years; today it is even hard to live up to 70. By the time people reach the age of 40 they are already on medications. This is because of our lifestyle and the food we eat. Even if we are sentenced to die eventually, we can still live healthy and better lives on earth as we serve God and humanity. This will happen only if we choose to follow God's way of healthy diets free from animal foods. We must eat vegetables, fruits, nuts, and grains, and exercise to build up our muscles and clean our body systems.

Remember, there is nothing your physician can do to cure irreversible heart disease caused by a bad lifestyle. It is evident that better health does not rely on better medicine, physicians, or hospitals. It relies on individual choice and lifestyle. It is also possible to change the way we perceive health and save ourselves from high costs for health care. It is a matter of choice. The word of God tells us, "I have set before you life and death, blessing and curse. Choose life so that you and your descendants may live" (Deuteronomy 30:15 NRSV).

Ellen White in her book *Ministry of Health* says, "In order to know what the best foods are, we must study God's original plan for man's diet. He who created man and who understands his needs, appointed Adam his foods. 'Behold he said I have given you every herb yielding seeds (fruits) ... and every tree in which is the fruit of a tree yielding seed: to you, it shall be for food'" (Genesis 3:18 ARV; White, 2007). God could have given them meat, but He did not. God wishes all human families to be healthy and happy. When we do not follow God's health rules and eat and drink as we please, we suffer from our choices.

There is no one to blame but ourselves. For many of us who are called to serve God and man on earth, we are reminded that our body is God's temple; we cannot eat and drink as we please. By not making the right choices when we know them, we dishonor our creator. Consequences of our choices may follow us throughout our lives. If we follow God's healthy diet, God will protect us from the diseases that affect others who do not follow God's ways.

Many of us do not have discipline about what we eat, and we may suffer from diseases that affect everyone else. We would have remained healthy and free from stress and heart disease if we had obeyed God's health laws. Our happy hearts would work as medicine to our souls. Proverbs 17:22 says, "A cheerful heart is good medicine but a downcast spirit dries up the bones" (NRSV).

In conclusion, please bear in mind that I am not in a position to stop you from taking heart, cholesterol, or diabetic medications. If you are taking these medications, you may depend on them for survival. I would encourage you to keep taking your medications until you're ready to change the lifestyle that is causing you to need the medication.

Your physician will be the one to lead you through those steps. What I am advocating in this book is to prevent heart disease, diabetes, and high cholesterol from happening in the first place, so you do not need medications.

As we have taken this scientific journey together in the book, you can see that my emphasis has been to point out the scientific proof to you as well as encouraging you to rethink health awareness and seek a better healthy life for you and your family. Avoid nonessential beverages and foods that may harm your body in the long run. Your body was made special by your Maker. It is not a garbage dumpster for anything you can put in your mouth.

God gave us good foods for better health (whole foods and unrefined vegetables and fruits). Humans made refined foods that cause health impairments. It is true that some people would rather eat fast food that is tasty, rather than thinking about what the food can do to their bodies. Most cases of heart disease, diabetes, and obesity are caused by how we eat and live.

Smoking cigarettes or other substances is an unnecessary habit that triggers heart problems and cancer. It is like working hard for your money and then buying poison to kill yourself. Smoking kills people who smoke and those around them. So much money is spent to try to cure the effects of smoking, yet when the lungs are damaged, there is nothing your physician can do to change your situation. It appears that the chemicals in these smoking substances are sometimes stronger than the mind. The solution to the problem of smoking is not to smoke at all; there is nothing good in smoking.

To those of us with this knowledge of healthy lifestyles, much is given, and much is required from us to live as an example to our families, friends, and patients. If we disregard our knowledge and assume that everything is and will be okay, we may pay a high price with our health. It makes no sense for a physician to recommend stopping smoking while he/she continues to drink unhealthy beverages and eat unhealthy foods. Let us practice what we preach.

REFERENCES

Aasum E, Hafstad AD, Severson DL, Larsen TS. Age-dependent changes in metabolism, contractile function, and ischemic sensitivity in hearts from db/db mice. *Diabetes.* 2003;52(2):434–441.

Abordo EA, Thornalley PJ. Synthesis and secretion of tumour necrosis factor-alpha by human monocytic THP-1 cells and chemotaxis induced by human serum albumin derivatives modified with methylglyoxal and glucose-derived advanced glycation endproducts. *Immunol Lett.* 1997;58(3):139–147.

Addis P. *Food and Nutrition News.* March/April 1990;62(2):7–10.

Alfin-Slater RB, Aftergood L. Lipids. In RS Goodhart, ME Shils, eds. *Modern Nutrition in Health and Disease.* 6th ed. Philadelphia: Lea and Febiger; 1980.

Allo SN, Lincoln TM, Wilson GL, Green FJ, Watanabe AM, Schaffer SW. Non-insulin-dependent diabetes-induced defects in cardiac cellular calcium regulation. *Am J Physiol.* 1991;260 (6 Pt 1): C1165–C1171.

American Society of Nuclear Cardiology. Five things physicians and patients should question. Available at: http://choosingwisely.org/wp-content/uploads/2012/04/5things_12_factsheet_Amer_Soc_Nuc_Cardio.pdf. Accessed August 17, 2012.

Andraws R, Berger JS, Brown DL. Effects of antibiotic therapy on outcomes of patients with coronary artery disease: a meta-analysis of randomized controlled trials. *JAMA* 2005;293(21):2641–2647. doi:10.1001/jama.293.21.2641. PMID 15928286.

Angelucci MEM, Cesário C, Hiroi RH, Rosalen PL, Da Cunha C. Effects of caffeine on learning and memory in rats tested in the Morris water maze. *Brazilian Journal of Medical and Biological Research.* 2002;35(10):1201–1208.

Arad Y, Goodman KJ, Roth M, Newstein D, Guerci AD. Coronary calcification, coronary disease risk factors, C-reactive protein, and atherosclerotic cardiovascular disease events: the St. Francis Heart Study. *J Am Coll Cardiol.* 2005;46(1):158–165.

Arnold ME, Petros TV, Beckwith GC, Gorman N. The effects of caffeine, impulsivity, and sex on memory for word lists. *Physiology & Behavior.* 1987;41(1):25–30.

Aso Y, Inukai T, Tayama K, Takemura Y. Serum concentrations of advanced glycation endproducts are associated with the development of atherosclerosis as well as diabetic microangiopathy in patients with type 2 diabetes. *Acta Diabetol.* 2000;37(2):87–92.

Avogaro A, Vigili de Kreutzenberg S, Negut C, Tiengo A, Scognamiglio R. Diabetic cardiomyopathy: a metabolic perspective. *Am J Cardiol.* 2004;93(8A).

Barnes B, Galton L. *Hyperthyroidism: The Unsuspected Illness.* New York: T Y Crowell: 1976.

Beamer AD, Lee TH, Cook EF, et al. Diagnostic implications for myocardial ischemia of the circadian variation of the onset of chest pain. *Am J Cardiol.* 1987;60(13):998–1002.

Berger JP, Buclin T, Haller E, Van Melle G, Yersin B. Right arm involvement and pain extension can help to differentiate coronary diseases from chest pain of other origin: a prospective emergency ward study of 278 consecutive patients admitted for chest pain. *J Intern Med.* 1990;227(3):165–172.

Bernstein GA, Carroll ME, Dean NW, Crosby RD, Perwien AR, Benowitz NL. Caffeine withdrawal in normal school-age children. *Journal of the American Academy of Child & Adolescent Psychiatry.* 1998;37(8):858–865.

Bing RJ, Siegel A, Ungar I, Gilbert M. Metabolism of the human heart: II. Studies on fat, ketone and amino acid metabolism. American Journal of Medicine. 1954;16(4):504–515.

Boie ET. Initial evaluation of chest pain. Emerg Med Clin North Am. 2005;23(4):937–957.

Brown A. *Emergency Medicine Diagnosis and Management.* 6th ed. 2011.

Buchanan J, Mazumder PK, Hu P, et al. Reduced cardiac efficiency and altered substrate metabolism precedes the onset of hyperglycemia and contractile dysfunction in two mouse models of insulin resistance and obesity. *Endocrinology.* 2005;146(12): 5341–5349.

Buse JB, Ginsberg HN, Bakris GL, et al. Primary prevention of cardiovascular diseases in people with diabetes mellitus: a scientific statement from the American Heart Association and the American Diabetes Association. *Circulation.* 2007;115(1):114–126. doi:10.1161/ CIRCULATIONAHA.106.179294.

Cannon CP, McCabe CH, Stone PH, et al. Circadian variation in the onset of unstable angina and non-Q-wave acute myocardial infarction (the TIMI III Registry and TIMI IIIB). *Am J Cardiol.* 1997;79(3):253–258.

Canto JG, Goldberg RJ, Hand MM, et al. Symptom presentation of women with acute coronary syndromes: myth vs reality. *Arch Intern Med.* 2007;167(22):2405–2413.

Centers for Disease Control and Prevention. Disparities in adult awareness of heart attack warning signs and symptoms—14 states, 2005. *MMWR.* 2008;57(7):175–179.

Centers for Disease Control and Prevention. Million hearts: strategies to reduce the prevalence of leading cardiovascular disease risk factors. United States, 2011.

Centers for Disease Control and Prevention. State specific mortality from sudden cardiac death: United States, 1999. *MMWR.* 2002;51(6):123–126.

Cesario DA, Brar R, Shivkumar K. Alterations in ion channel physiology in diabetic cardiomyopathy. *Endocrinol Metab Clin North Am.* 2006;35(3):601–610.

Charonis AS, Reger LA, Dege JE, et al. Laminin alterations after in vitro nonenzymatic glycosylation. *Diabetes.* 1990;39(7):807–814. doi:10.2337/diabetes.39.7.807. PMID 2113013.

Chatham JC, Forder JR. Relationship between cardiac function and substrate oxidation in hearts of diabetic rats. *Am J Physiol.* 1997;273(1 Pt 2).

Chatham JC, Gao ZP, Bonen A, Forder JR. Preferential inhibition of lactate oxidation relative to glucose oxidation in the rat heart following diabetes. *Cardiovascular Research.* 1999;43(1):96–106.

Choi KM, Zhong Y, Hoit BD, et al. Defective intracellular Ca2+signaling contributes to cardiomyopathy in Type 1 diabetic rats. *Am J Physiol Heart Circ Physiol.* 2002;283(4): H1398–H1408. doi:10.1152/ajpheart.00313.2002.

Clarke R, Halsey J, Bennett D, Lewington S. Homocysteine and vascular disease: review of published results of the homocysteine-lowering trials. *J Inherit Metab Dis.* 2011;34(1):83–91.

Clerk LH, Rattigan S, Clark MG. Lipid infusion impairs physiologic insulin-mediated capillary recruitment and muscle glucose uptake in vivo. *Diabetes.* 2002;51.

Clevidence BA, et al. Plasma lipoprotein (a) levels in men and women consuming diets enriched in saturated, cis-, or trans-monounsaturated fatty acids. *Arterioscler Thromb Vasc Biol.* 1997;17:1657-166.

Cohen LA, et al. Dietary fat and mammary cancer. II. Modulation of serum and tumor lipid composition and tumor prostaglandins by different dietary fats: association with tumor incidence patterns. *J Natl Cancer Inst.* 1986;77:43.

Dahlen GH, et al. The importance of serum lipoprotein (a) as an independent risk factor for premature coronary artery disease in middle-aged black and white women from the United States. *J Intern Med.* Nov 1998;244(5):417–424.

D'Aiuto F, Parkar M, Nibali L, Suvan J, Lessem J, Tonetti MS. Periodontal infections cause changes in traditional and novel cardiovascular risk factors: results from a randomized controlled clinical trial. *Am Heart J.* 2006;151(5):977–984.

Davis TM, Fortun P, Mulder J, Davis WA, Bruce DG. Silent myocardial infarction and its prognosis in a community-based cohort of Type 2 diabetic patients: the Fremantle Diabetes Study. *Diabetologia.* 2004;47(3):395–399.

Davis TM, Balme M, Jackson D, Stuccio G, Bruce DG. The diagonal ear lobe crease (Frank's sign) is not associated with coronary artery disease or retinopathy in type 2 diabetes: the Fremantle Diabetes Study. *Aust N Z J Med.* 2000;30(5):573–577.

Devlin RJ, Henry JA. Clinical review: Major consequences of illicit drug consumption. *Crit Care*. 2008;12(1):202. doi:10.1186/cc6166.

Dohi T, Daida H (April 2010). [Change of concept and pathophysiology in acute coronary syndrome]. *Nippon Rinsho* (in Japanese). 2010;68(4):592–596.

Engelberg H. Low serum cholesterol and suicide. *Lancet*. March 21, 1992;339:727–728.

Enig MG. *Trans Fatty Acids in the Food Supply: A Comprehensive Report Covering 60 Years of Research*. 2nd ed. Silver Spring, MD: Enig Associates; 1995.

Enig MG, et al. Dietary fat and cancer trends—a critique. *Fed Proc*. July 1978;37(9):2215–2220.

Erhardt L, Herlitz J, Bossaert L, et al. Task force on the management of chest pain. *Eur Heart J*. 2002;23(15):1153–1176.

Erikson G, Hager L, Houseworth C, Dungan J, Petros T, Beckwith B. The effects of caffeine on memory for word lists. *Physiology & Behavior*. 1985;35:47–51.

Fallon S, Enig MG. Diet and heart disease—not what you think. *Consumers' Research*. July 1996;15–19.

Ferri C, Piccoli A, Laurenti O, et al. Atrial atriuretic factor in hypertensive and normotensive diabetic patients. *Diabetes Care*. 1994;17(3):195–200.

Finck BN, Han X, Courtois M, et al. A critical role for PPARalpha-mediated lipotoxicity in the pathogenesis of diabetic cardiomyopathy: modulation by dietary fat content. *Proceedings of the National Academy of Sciences of the United States of America*. 2003;100(3):1226–1231.

Fonarow GC, Srikanthan P. Diabetic cardiomyopathy. *Endocrinol Metab Clin North Am.* 2006;35(3):575–599.

Graham I, Atar D, Borch-Johnsen K, et al. European guidelines on cardiovascular disease prevention in clinical practice: executive summary: Fourth Joint Task Force of the European Society of Cardiology and Other Societies on Cardiovascular Disease Prevention in Clinical Practice (Constituted by representatives of nine societies and by invited experts). *Eur Heart J.* 2007;28(19).

Greenland P, LaBree L, Azen SP, Doherty TM, Detrano RC. Coronary artery calcium score combined with Framingham score for risk prediction in asymptomatic individuals. *JAMA.* 2004;291(2):210–215.

Grishman A. New type of cardiomyopathy associated with diabetic glomerulosclerosis. *Am J Cardiol.* 1972;30(6):595–602.

Giardino I, Edelstein D, Brownlee M. Nonenzymatic glycosylation in vitro and in bovine endothelial cells alters basic fibroblast growth factor activity. A model for intracellular glycosylation in diabetes. *J Clin Invest.* 1994;94(1):110–117.

Golfman LS, Wilson CR, Sharma S, et al. Activation of PPA Rgamma enhances myocardial glucose oxidation and improves contractile function in isolated working hearts of ZDF rats. *Am J Physiol Endocrinol Metab.* 2005;289(2):E328–E336.

Hameleers P, Van Boxtel M, Hogervorst E, Riedel W, Houx P, Buntinx F, Jolles J. Habitual caffeine consumption and its relation to memory, attention, planning capacity and psychomotor performance across multiple age groups. *Hum Psychopharmacol.* 2000;15(8):573–581.

Hamm CW, Bassand JP, Agewall S, et al. ESC Guidelines for the management of acute coronary syndromes in patients presenting without persistent ST-segment elevation: The Task Force for the management of acute coronary syndromes (ACS) in patients presenting without persistent

ST-segment elevation of the European Society of Cardiology (ESC). *Eur Heart J.* 2011;32(23):2999–3054.

Heidenreich PA, Trogdon JG, Khavjou OA, et al. Forecasting the future of cardiovascular disease in the United States: a policy statement from the American Heart Association. *Circulation.* 2011;123:933–944.

Heron M. Deaths: Leading causes for 2008. Available at: http://www.cdc.gov/nchs/data/nvsr/nvsr60/nvsr60_06.pdf.

Herz R. Caffeine effects on mood and memory. *Behav Res Ther.* 1999;37(9): 869–879.

Higuchi M, Miyagi K, Nakasone J, Sakanashi M. Role of high glycogen in underperfused diabetic rat hearts with added norepinephrine. *J Cardiovasc Pharmacol.* 1995;26(6):899–907.

Hogervorst E, et al. Caffeine improves memory performance during distraction in middle-aged, but not in young or old subjects. *Human Psychopharmacology: Clinical and Experimental.* 1998;13(4):277–284.

Holman, RT. *Geometrical and Positional Fatty Acid Isomers.* Champaign, IL: American Oil Chemists' Society; 1979.

Hubert H, et al. Obesity as an independent risk factor for cardiovascular disease: a 26-year follow-up of participants in the Framingham Heart Study. *Circulation.* 1983;67:968.

JAMA. Multiple risk factor intervention trial; risk factor changes and mortality results. *JAMA.* September 24, 1982; 248(12):1465.

Janket SJ, Baird AE, Chuang SK, Jones JA. Meta-analysis of periodontal disease and risk of coronary heart disease and stroke. *Oral Surg Oral Med Oral Pathol Oral Radiol Endod.* 2003;95(5):559–569.

Jensen G, Nyboe J, Appleyard M, Schnohr P. Risk factors for acute myocardial infarction in Copenhagen, II: Smoking, alcohol intake, physical activity, obesity, oral contraception, diabetes, lipids, and blood pressure. *Eur Heart J.* 1991;12(3):298–308.

Jourdon P, Feuvray D. Calcium and potassium currents in ventricular myocytes isolated from diabetic rats. *J Physiol. (Lond.)* 1993;470:411–429.

Kabara, JJ. *The Pharmacological Effects of Lipids.* Champaign, IL: American Oil Chemists' Society; 1978.

Kannel WB. Silent myocardial ischemia and infarction: insights from the Framingham Study. *Cardiol Clin.* 1986;4(4):583–591.

Karvounis HI, Papadopoulos CE, Zaglavara TA, et al. Evidence of left ventricular dysfunction in asymptomatic elderly patients with non-insulin-dependent diabetes mellitus. *Angiology.* 2004;55(5):549–555.

Khosla P, Hayes KC. Dietary trans-monounsaturated fatty acids negatively impact plasma lipids in humans: critical review of the evidence. *J Am Coll Nutr.* 1996;15:325–339.

Kivimäki M, Nyberg ST, Batty GD, et al. Job strain as a risk factor for coronary heart disease: a collaborative meta-analysis of individual participant data. *Lancet.* 2012;380(9852):1491–1497.

Kochanek KD, Xu JQ, Murphy SL, Miniño AM, Kung HC. Deaths: final data for 2009. Available at: http://www.cdc.gov/nchs/data/nvsr/nvsr60/nvsr60_03.pdf

Koga Y, et al. Recent trends in cardiovascular disease and risk factors in the seven countries study: Japan. In *Lessons for Science from the Seven Countries Study,* H Toshima et al., eds. New York: Springer; 1994, 63–74.

Kosuge M, Kimura K, Ishikawa T, et al. Differences between men and women in terms of clinical features of ST-segment elevation acute myocardial infarction. *Circulation Journal*. 2006;70(3):222–226.

Krijnen PA, Nijmeijer R, Meijer CJ, Visser CA, Hack CE, Niessen HW. Apoptosis in myocardial ischaemia and infarction. *J Clin Pathol*. 2002;55(11):801–811.

Koya D, King GL. Protein kinase C activation and the development of diabetic complications. *Diabetes*. 1998;47(6):859–866.

Lackland DT, et al. The need for accurate nutrition survey methodology: the South Carolina experience. *J Nutr*. 1990;120:11S:1433–1436.

Lawson, LD, Kummerow F. Beta-oxidation of the coenzyme A esters of vaccenic, elaidic, and petroselaidic acids by rat heart mitochondria. *Lipids*. 1979;14:501–503.

Lee AY, Chung SS. Contributions of polyol pathway to oxidative stress in diabetic cataract. *FASEB J*. 1999;13(1):23–30.

Lesk VE, Womble SP. Caffeine, priming, and tip of the tongue: evidence for plasticity in the phonological system. *Behavioural Neuroscience*. 2004;118(3):453–461.Little RA, Frayn KN, Randall PE, et al. Plasma catecholamines in the acute phase of the response to myocardial infarction. *Arch Emerg Med*. 1986;3(1):20–27.

Li SH, McNeill JH. In vivo effects of vanadium on GLUT4 translocation in cardiac tissue of STZ-diabetic rats. *Mol Cell Biochem*. 2001;217(1-2):121–129.

Lonn E. Homocysteine in the prevention of ischemic heart disease, stroke and venous thromboembolism: therapeutic target or just another distraction? *Curr Opin Hematol*. 2007; 14(5):481–487.

Luszczki JJ, Zuchora M, Kozinska J, Ozog AA. Caffeine impairs long-term memory in the step-through passive avoidance task in mice. *Annales Universitatis Mariae Curie-Sklodowska.* 2006.

Magyar J, Cseresnyés Z, Rusznák Z, Sipos I, Szücs G, Kovács L. Effects of insulin on potassium currents of rat ventricular myocytes in streptozotocin diabetes. *Gen Physiol Biophys.* 1995;14(3):191–201.

Makino N, Dhalla KS, Elimban V, Dhalla NS. Sarcolemmal Ca2+ transport in streptozotocin-induced diabetic cardiomyopathy in rats. *Am J Physiol.* 1987;253(2 Pt 1):E202–E207.

Mallinson, T. Myocardial infarction. *Focus on First Aid.* 2010;15:15.

Marcus GM, Cohen J, Varosy PD, et al. The utility of gestures in patients with chest discomfort. *Am J Med.* 2007;120(1):83–89.

Mayo Clinic. Caffeine content for coffee, tea, soda, and more. Available at: http://www.mayoclinic.com/health/caffeine/AN01211. Accessed October 15, 2012.

McSweeney JC, Cody M, O'Sullivan P, Elberson K, Moser DK, Garvin BJ. Women's early warning symptoms of acute myocardial infarction. *Circulation.* 2003;108(21):2619–2623.

Mitchell PJ. (1992). Effects of caffeine, time of day and user history on study-related performance. *Psychopharmacology.* 1992;109(1-2):121–126.

Moe KT, Wong P. Current trends in diagnostic biomarkers of acute coronary syndrome. *Ann Acad Med Singapore.* 2010;39(3):210–215.

Moore TJ. *Lifespan: What Really Affects Human Longevity.* New York: Simon and Schuster; 1990.

Mulder G, Visscher B. (1930). The carbohydrate metabolism of the heart. *American Journal of Physiology.* 1930;94:630–640.

Muller JE, Stone PH, Turi ZG, et al. Circadian variation in the frequency of onset of acute myocardial infarction. *N Engl J Med.* 1985;313(21):1315–1322.

Nyboe J, Jensen G, Appleyard M, Schnohr P. Risk factors for acute myocardial infarction in Copenhagen. I: Hereditary, educational and socioeconomic factors. Copenhagen City Heart Study. *Eur Heart J.* 1989;10(10):910–916.

O'Connor RE, Brady W, Brooks SC, et al. Part 10: acute coronary syndromes: 2010 American Heart Association Guidelines for Cardiopulmonary Resuscitation and Emergency Cardiovascular Care. *Circulation.* 2010;122(18 Suppl 3):S787–S817. doi: 10.1161/ CIRCULATIONAHA.110.971028.

Oliver MF, Opie LH. Effects of glucose and fatty acids on myocardial ischaemia and arrhythmias. *Lancet.* 1994;343(8890):155–158.

Pereira L, Matthes J, Schuster I, et al. Mechanisms of [Ca2+] i transient decrease in cardiomyopathy of db/db type 2 diabetic mice. *Diabetes.* 2006;55(3):608–615.

Pinckney ER, Pinckney C. *The Cholesterol Controversy.* Los Angeles, CA: Sherbourne Press; 1973.

Price W. *Nutrition and Physical Degeneration.* San Diego, CA: Price-Pottenger Nutrition Foundation; 1945.

Reznik AG. [Morphology of acute myocardial infarction at prenecrotic stage]. *Kardiologiia* (in Russian). 2010;50(1):4–8.

Richardson NJ, Elliman NA, Rogers PJ. Mood and performance effects of caffeine in relation to acute and chronic caffeine deprivation. *Pharmacology Biochemistry and Behaviour.* 1995;52(2):313–320.

Roe MT, Messenger JC, Weintraub WS, et al. Treatments, trends, and outcomes of acute myocardial infarction and percutaneous coronary intervention. *J Am Coll Cardiol*. 2010;56(4):254–263. doi: 10.1016/j.jacc.2010.05.008.

Roger VL, Go AS, Lloyd-Jones DM, et al. Heart disease and stroke statistics—2012 update: a report from the American Heart Association. *Circulation*. 2012;125(1):e2–e220. doi: 10.1161/CIR.0b013e31823ac046.

Rogers PJ, Heatherley SV, Hayward RC, Seers HE, Hill J, Kane M. Effects of caffeine and caffeine withdrawal on mood and cognitive performance degraded by sleep deprivation. *Psychopharmacology*. 2005;179(4):742–752.

Rubin R, Strayer DS, eds. *Rubin's Pathology: Clinicopathological Foundations of Medicine*. Maryland: Lippincott Williams & Wilkins.

Ruddy TD, Shumak SL, Liu PP, et al. The relationship of cardiac diastolic dysfunction to concurrent hormonal and metabolic status in type I diabetes mellitus. *J Clin Endocrinol Metab*. 1988;66(1):113–118.

Ryan L, Hatfield C, Hofstetter M. Caffeine reduces time-of-day effects on memory performance in older adults. *Psychol Sci*. 2002;13(1):68–71.

Scannapieco FA, Bush RB, Paju S. Associations between periodontal disease and risk for atherosclerosis, cardiovascular disease, and stroke. A systematic review. *Ann Periodontol*. 2003;8(1):38–53.

Schmitt JA, et al. Memory functions and focused attention in middle-aged and elderly subjects are unaffected by a low, acute dose of caffeine. *J Nutr Health Aging*. 2003;7(5):301–303.

Severson DL. Diabetic cardiomyopathy: recent evidence from mouse models of type 1 and type 2 diabetes. *Can J Physiol Pharmacol*. 2004;82(10):813–823.

Smith MM, Lifshitz F. Excess fruit juice consumption as a contributing factor in nonorganic failure to thrive. *Pediatrics.* 1994;93(3):438–443.

Smith R, Pinckney ER. *Diet, Blood Cholesterol and Coronary Heart Disease: A Critical Review of the Literature.* Vol. 2. Sherman Oaks, CA: Vector Enterprises; 1991.

Spaan J, Kolyva C, van den Wijngaard J, et al. Coronary structure and perfusion in health and disease. *Philos Trans A Math Phys Eng Sci.* 2008;366(1878):3137–3153. doi: 10.1098/rsta.2008.0075.

Stanley WC, Recchia FA, Lopaschuk GD. Myocardial substrate metabolism in the normal and failing heart. *Physiol Rev.* 2005;85(3):1093–1129.

Steptoe A, Kivimäki M. Stress and cardiovascular disease. *Nat Rev Cardiol.* 2012;9(6):360-370. doi: 10.1038/nrcardio.2012.45.

Suga H. Ventricular energetics. *Physiol Rev.* 1990;70(2):247–277.

Terry W, Phifer B. Caffeine and memory performance on the AVLT. *J Clin Psychol.* 1986;42(6):860–863.

Teshima Y, Takahashi N, Saikawa T, et al. Diminished expression of sarcoplasmic reticulum Ca2+-ATPase and ryanodine sensitive Ca2+Channel mRNA in streptozotocin-induced diabetic rat heart. *J Mol Cell Cardiol.* 2000;32(4):655–664.

Thygesen K, Alpert JS, White HD. Universal definition of myocardial infarction. *Eur Heart J.* 2007;28(20):2525–2538.

Tsujita K, Kaikita K, Soejima H, Sugiyama S, Ogawa H. [Acute coronary syndrome-initiating factors]. *Nippon Rinsho* (in Japanese). 2010;68(4):607–614.

Ungar I, Gilbert M, Siegel A, Blain JM, Bing RJ. Studies on myocardial metabolism. IV. Myocardial metabolism in diabetes. *Am J Med.* 1955;18(3):385–396.

Valensi P, Lorgis L, Cottin Y. Prevalence, incidence, predictive factors and prognosis of silent myocardial infarction: a review of the literature. *Arch Cardiovasc Dis.* 2011;104(3):178–188. doi: 10.1016/j.acvd.2010.11.013.

Van Boxtel MPJ, Schmitt JAJ. Age-related changes in the effects of coffee on memory and cognitive performance. In Nehlig A, ed. *Coffee, Tea, Chocolate, and the Brain.* CRC Press; 2004.

Van de Werf F, Bax J, Betriu A, et al. Management of acute myocardial infarction in patients presenting with persistent ST-segment elevation: the Task Force on the Management of ST-Segment Elevation Acute Myocardial Infarction of the European Society of Cardiology. *Eur Heart J.* 2008;29(23):2909–2945. doi: 10.1093/eurheartj/ehn416.

Warburton DM. Effects of caffeine on cognition and mood without caffeine abstinence. *Psychopharmacology.* 1995;119(1):66–70.

Warburton DM, Bersellinni E, Sweeney E. An evaluation of a caffeinated taurine drink on mood, memory and information processing in healthy volunteers without caffeine abstinence. *Psychopharmacology.* 2001;158(3):322–328.

Warren-Gash C, Smeeth L, Hayward AC. Influenza as a trigger for acute myocardial infarction or death from cardiovascular disease: a systematic review. *Lancet Infect Dis.* 2009;9(10):601–610. doi: 10.1016/S1473-3099(09)70233-6.

Watkins BA, et al. *Importance of Vitamin E in Bone Formation and in Chrondrocyte Function.* Lafayette, IN: AOCS Proceedings; 1996.

Watkins BA, Seifert MF. Food lipids and bone health. In McDonald RE, Min DB, eds. *Food Lipids and Health.* New York: Marcel Dekker; 1996.

White E. *Ministry of Healing*. Atamont, TN: Harvesttime Books; 2007.

White BC, Lincoln CA, Pearce NW, Reeb R, Vaida C. Anxiety and muscle tension as consequences of caffeine withdrawal. *Science*. 1980;209(4464):1547–1548.

Wilson AM, Ryan MC, Boyle AJ. The novel role of C-reactive protein in cardiovascular disease: risk marker or pathogen. *Int J Cardiol*. 2006;106(3):291–297.

Wold LE, Dutta K, Mason MM, et al. Impaired SERCA function contributes to cardiomyocyte dysfunction in insulin resistant rats. *J Mol Cell Cardiol*. 2005;39(2):297–307.

Wood WG, et al. Recent advances in brain cholesterol dynamics: transport, domains, and Alzheimer's disease. *Lipids*. 1999;34(3):225–234.

Woollard KJ, Geissmann F. Monocytes in atherosclerosis: subsets and functions. *Nat Rev Cardiol*. 2010;7(2):77–86. doi: 10.1038/nrcardio.2009.228.

World Health Organization. *The Global Burden of Disease: 2004 Update*. Geneva: World Health Organization; 2008.

Yaras N, Ugur M, Ozdemir S, et al. Effects of diabetes on ryanodine receptor Ca release channel (RyR2) and Ca2+ homeostasis in rat heart. *Diabetes*. 2005;54(11):3082–3088.

Zhao XY, Hu SJ, Li J, Mou Y, Chen BP, Xia Q. Decreased cardiac sarcoplasmic reticulum Ca2+ -ATPase activity contributes to cardiac dysfunction in streptozotocin-induced diabetic rats. *J Physiol Biochem*. 2006;62(1):1–8.

Zhou YT, Grayburn P, Karim A, et al. Lipotoxic heart disease in obese rats: implications for human obesity. *Proc Natl Acad Sci U S A*. 2000;97(4):1784–1789.

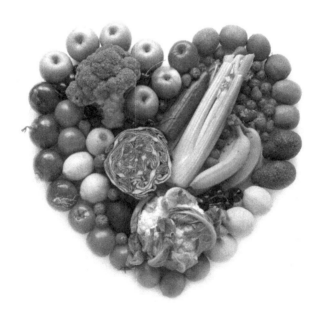